Reflective Practice in Nursing

Fifth Edition

Edited by

Chris Bulman
PhD, MSc, BSc (Hons), RN, RNT, PGCEA
Senior Lecturer, Faculty of Health and Life Sciences,
Oxford Brookes University, Oxford, UK

Sue Schutz
MSc, RGN, Cert Ed (FE)
Senior Lecturer, Faculty of Health and Life Sciences,
Oxford Brookes University, Oxford;
Part-time PhD Student,
University of Southampton, Southampton, UK

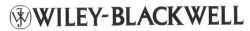

WILEY-BLACKWELL

A John Wiley & Sons, Ltd., Publication

Registered Office
John Wiley & Sons, Ltd, The Atrium, Southern Gate, Chichester, West Sussex, PO19 8SQ, UK

Editorial Offices
9600 Garsington Road, Oxford, OX4 2DQ, UK
The Atrium, Southern Gate, Chichester, West Sussex, PO19 8SQ, UK
111 River Street, Hoboken, NJ 07030-5774, USA

For details of our global editorial offices, for customer services and for information about how to apply for permission to reuse the copyright material in this book please see our website at www.wiley.com/wiley-blackwell.

Library of Congress Cataloging-in-Publication Data

Reflective practice in nursing / edited by Chris Bulman, Sue Schutz. – 5th ed.
  p. ; cm.
 Includes bibliographical references and index.
 ISBN 978-0-470-65810-9 (pbk. : alk. paper)
I. Bulman, Chris. II. Schutz, Sue. [DNLM: 1. Nursing. 2. Education, Nursing.
3. Learning. 4. Nursing Process. 5. Philosophy, Nursing. 6. Thinking. WY 16]
  610.73–dc23
                                          2012032716

A catalogue record for this book is available from the British Library.

Wiley also publishes its books in a variety of electronic formats. Some content that appears in print may not be available in electronic books.

Cover image: iStock image 19247374
Cover design by Sophie Ford www.hisandhersdesign.co.uk

Set in 10/12pt Avenir by SPi Publisher Services, Pondicherry, India
Printed and bound in Malaysia by Vivar Printing Sdn Bhd

3   2015

Contents

List of Contributors

Sue Atkins MSc, RN, RM, Dip Nursing, Dip Nursing Ed, Senior Lecturer, Faculty of Health and Life Sciences, Oxford Brookes University, Oxford, UK

Chris Bulman PhD, MSc, BSc (Hons), RN, RNT, PGCEA, Senior Lecturer, Faculty of Health and Life Sciences, Oxford Brookes University, Oxford, UK

Bernadette Carter PhD, PGCE, BSc, RSCN, SRN, Professor of Children's Nursing, Families, Children and Life Transitions Research Group, Department of Nursing, University of Central Lancashire, Preston, UK

Paul Cassedy RMN, RNT, MA Counselling Practice, Health Lecturer, School of Nursing, University of Nottingham, Nottingham, UK

John Driscoll BSc (Hons) Nursing, DPSN, Cert Ed (FE), RGN, RMN, Freelance CPD Consultant and Coach, Norfolk, UK

Sue Duke PhD, MSc, BSc, PGDE, RN, RNT, Consultant Practitioner in Cancer and Palliative Care, Senior Lecturer, Faculty of Health Sciences, University of Southampton, Southampton, UK

Charlotte Maddison MSc, BA (Hons), RGN, PGCE, Senior Lecturer, Faculty of Health and Life Sciences, Oxford Brookes University, Oxford, UK

Sue Schutz MSc, RGN, Cert Ed (FE), Senior Lecturer, Faculty of Health and Life Sciences, Oxford Brookes University, Oxford; Part-time PhD Student, University of Southampton, Southampton, UK

Pam Sharp MSc, PG Dip, RGN, Senior Lecturer, Faculty of Health and Life Sciences, Oxford Brookes University, Oxford, UK

Sylvina Tate   MSc, PGDE, BSc (Hons), Dip Nursing (London), RGN, ENB 998, BTech Certificates Massage and Aromatherapy, Dru Yoga Teachers Diploma, Reiki II Practitioner Certificate, Life Coach, formerly Principal Lecturer, School of Life Sciences, University of Westminster, London, UK

Preface

Welcome to the fifth edition of *Reflective Practice in Nursing*. This new edition responds to the interest in reflective practice amongst nurses and offers a motivating and accessible text about reflection. Fundamentally, this book does not assume any previous knowledge about reflection and aims to be useful to those wanting to learn about what it has to offer them. Past editions of *Reflective Practice in Nursing* have appealed to a wide variety of readers – undergraduate and postgraduate students, practitioners from a range of backgrounds and experience, plus teachers, managers, mentors and professionals from other disciplines. This past success has motivated us to produce this latest publication.

The fifth edition has much new to offer. The extensively updated first chapter introduces you to reflection in relation to the current issues that affect nursing. The chapter considers some philosophical underpinnings, plus some of the 'dangers' of reflection and the role reflection can play in the evidence-based practice movement. It looks at other key issues including communicating practice knowledge, empowerment and change, knowledge tensions and the relevance of reflection to nurse education and practice. The chapter on skills for reflection has also been updated and includes a valuable exploration of the attributes of the reflective practitioner.

A new chapter on writing reflectively offers some inspiring and uplifting guidance and introduces the idea of reflective writing as a method of deep, self-directed learning. An extensively updated chapter on group reflection offers plenty of advice and tips for practitioners and educationalists, as well as a lively critique of the current literature. The chapter on the student's and mentor's journey into reflection focuses on pre-registration students and the preparation and support of mentors. The chapter deliberates some of the contemporary issues that affect nurses' and mentors' capacities to develop and use reflection. The chapter illustrates how the development and use of reflection is valuable to nurses' and mentors' personal development and the ongoing achievement of thoughtful and excellent professional practice.

The chapter focusing on clinical supervision in nursing is another exciting new addition to this book. It draws on the experiences and knowledge of two highly experienced supervisors and considers the issues around supervision for supervisors. A new chapter on a personal exploration of reflection and clinical expertise adds to those contributed by Sue Duke to past editions of this book and offers some controversial and essential 'food for thought' concerning being a reflective practitioner in nursing today. The chapter on assessing and evaluating reflection remains and has been added to and updated. This is a challenging area for debate but remains one that we feel needs to be raised, if practice knowledge is to be valued in the same way as theoretical knowledge. Finally, the last chapter gives an extensively revised guide to getting started with reflection, drawing on other areas of the book and giving more tips, cautions, helpful frameworks and new examples to help you to begin your journey with reflection.

In essence, our aim is to make you curious about reflection, in a spirit that gets you thinking about the issues involved and challenges you to look at your view of the world. Essentially, we hope it will be useful to all those involved and interested in developing, using and exploring reflective practice.

Chris Bulman and Sue Schutz
2012

Chapter 1
An introduction to reflection

Chris Bulman

Faculty of Health and Life Sciences, Oxford Brookes University, Oxford, UK

Introduction

Every contributor to this book is motivated by an interest in reflection. Within this fifth edition, we have presented experience, research and theory in order to help you get a better grasp of reflection, especially if you are considering it for the first time. This probably means that you are a student but you could equally be a supervisor, mentor or senior nurse furthering your understanding of reflection, or a nurse teacher interested in reflective education. Whilst this is a book that clearly advocates reflection, we are also aware of the difficulties and criticisms associated with it. Thus we offer a book that will give you some help with whatever journey you are taking with reflection, but will also get you thinking critically about the issues involved.

Contemporary challenges for reflective nursing practice and education

There is no doubt that reflection continues to be of interest to nurses and to influence nursing practice and education around the world. It remains a concept that I and fellow authors are committed to. We believe that being reflective is essential for effective and person-centred professional practice. Significantly, current financial concerns and pressures are affecting health services across many countries. This has had an impact on nursing education and frontline clinical services. It has unquestionably influenced the amount of time, energy and support that nurses have to constructively consider and learn from their practice. All this has affected learning opportunities, such as provision of clinical supervision for

Reflective Practice in Nursing, Fifth Edition. Edited by Chris Bulman and Sue Schutz.
© 2013 John Wiley & Sons, Ltd. Published 2013 by John Wiley & Sons, Ltd.

practitioners, time for informally reflecting with colleagues, and defending the relevance of reflective education for the development of clinical judgement, alongside the juggernaut which is evidence-based practice education. (I'll return to this later in the chapter.) With these current challenges in mind, we believe it is even more vital to continue to write about reflection as a positive way to learn from experience – warts and all!

Explaining the concept of reflection

Starting with Aristotle

Getting to grips with an explanation of reflection is a sensible place to start. The concept of reflection is not as new as you might imagine. At the outset, I will underline the influence of the Ancient Greek philosopher Aristotle and his notion of practical wisdom/judgement or *phronesis*. Aristotle emphasised the importance of reflecting in the 'real world' and developing experience of it. He emphasised the requirement to pay attention to emotions and imagination in order to develop our perception of the world, so that emotion and imagination are not relegated to unwanted self-indulgent urges or corrupting influences that get in the way of 'good' rational thinking, but rather are a responsive and elective part of our thinking. In this way, Aristotle believed it was possible to develop real practical insight, responsiveness and understanding (Nussbaum 1990). So you can begin to see how this might be related to the development of practical knowledge, considering how we feel, as well as think, about practice, and finding a way of communicating this sort of knowledge to others.

Dewey

The educationalist and philosopher John Dewey has been extremely influential in contemporary discussion about the concept of reflection. Dewey developed his ideas on thinking and learning and focused on the concept of thinking reflectively. He defined reflection as:

> 'Active, persistent and careful consideration of any belief or supposed form of knowledge in the light of the grounds that support it and the further conclusions to which it tends.' (Dewey 1933, p.9)

Dewey saw reflective thinking as thinking with a purpose and focused strongly on the need to test out and challenge true beliefs by applying the scientific method through deductive reasoning and experimentation. He implied that emotions and feelings are part of reflective thinking but, in contrast to Aristotle, this is not something that he expanded on. He made some important assumptions about people, emphasising our tendencies towards quick solutions, custom and 'mental ruts' and the pervading influence of culture and the environment upon our thinking:

> 'External monotony and internal routine are the worst enemies of wonder.' (Dewey 1933, p.52)

Dewey also emphasised the need for thinking to be directly linked with action, demonstrating the pragmatic nature of his philosophy, and suggested that any thinking can be intellectual, thus emphasising the importance of the practical as well as the theoretical. He has influenced the work of many others, for example, Clarke and Graham (1996), who have also helpfully described the complexity of experiences, and reflection as a reasoning out process.

> 'By engaging in reflection people are usually engaging in a period of thinking in order to examine often complex experiences or situations. The period of thinking (reflection) allows the individual to make sense of an experience, perhaps to liken the experience to other similar experiences and to place it in context. Faced with complex decisions, thinking it through (reflecting) allows the individual to separate out the various influencing factors and come to a reasoned decision or course of action.' (Clarke and Graham 1996, p.26)

Schön

The philosopher Donald Schön has been a huge influence on the development of reflection in professional education. Importantly, Schön (1983, 1987) believed that practice should be central to professional curricula; consequently he saw learning by 'doing' becoming the core of programmes rather than an add-on, with students investing in practice and time, in order to learn from it. This implies that students need to develop a commitment to practice and the motivation to learn from it (Bulman 2004).

Schön defined reflection-on-action as:

> '... thinking back on what we have done in order to discover how our knowing in action may have contributed to an unexpected outcome. We may do so after the fact, in tranquillity, or we may pause in the midst of action (stop and think).' (Schön 1987, p.26)

This focuses on retrospective critical thinking, to construct and reconstruct events in order to develop oneself as a practitioner and person. Significantly, his concept of reflection involves more than 'intellectual' thinking, since practitioners' feelings and an acknowledgement of an interrelationship with action are also important. (Can you see a link back to Aristotle's practical wisdom?) Yet Schön's work focused more on reflection-in-action which he saw as a distinguishing feature of expert practitioners who were able to experiment and think about their practice whilst they were doing it:

> '… where we may reflect in the midst of action without interrupting it. Our thinking serves to reshape what we are doing while we are doing it.' (Schön 1987, p.26)

As you can see, this is a different concept from reflection-on-action since it is not about carrying out a 'post mortem' (however speedy) on an experience but concerns thinking and knowing in the midst of action. Schön saw reflection-in-action as a distinguishing feature of expert practitioners who are able to experiment and think about their practice whilst they are doing it; this idea is fundamental to his theory of professional expertise. It is difficult to conceptualise, and you will find it is sometimes misrepresented by those who view reflection-on-action and reflection-in-action as the same. Essentially, it is a different concept to that explored in this book, which largely focuses on reflection concerned with the construction of knowledge after an experience and the teaching and learning associated with it.

Contemporary descriptions of reflection

Other authors' contributions are also useful in developing an appreciation of the concept of reflection. Wong et al. (1997) have described the central point of reflection on experience, with the trigger point of the process usually starting with an emotional response (Dewey 1933), which can be both positive (Boud et al. 1985) and uncomfortable (Atkins and Murphy 1993). More recently, Freshwater et al. (2008, p.4) have described reflection as retrospectively making sense of experience in order to influence future practice. Similarly, O'Donovan's (2007) research describes reflection as a process of deliberative thinking, looking back, examining oneself and one's practice in order to improve future practice. Like Clarke and Graham (1996), all these authors have described the reflective process as one of making sense of an experience and consequently learning from it.

The influence of critical theory

The use of reflection within professional practice and education has also been heavily influenced by critical theory stemming from the work of Habermas (1977) and the early work of such leading educationalists as Van Manen (1977), Mezirow (1981) and Brookfield (1987). Mulhall and Le May (1999) explain that critical theory enquiry argues that society is structured by meanings, rules and habits. Its purpose is to reveal aspects of society that confine human freedom and maintain the status quo. The theory's central contention is that each of us is located historically and socially, and consequently, objective knowledge is dismissed. You can see how critical theory has influenced the descriptions of influential authors below.

> 'Reflective learning is the process of internally examining and exploring an issue of concern, triggered by an experience, which creates and clarifies meaning in terms of self and which results in a changed conceptual perspective.' (Boyd and Fales 1983, p.113)

> 'Reflection in the context of learning is a generic term for those intellectual and affective activities in which individuals engage to explore their experiences in order to lead to new understandings and appreciations.' (Boud et al. 1985, p.19)

> 'I describe reflection as being mindful of self, either within or after experience, like a mirror to which the practitioner can view and focus self within the context of a particular experience, in order to confront, understand and move toward resolving contradiction between one's vision and actual practice. Through the conflict of contradiction, the commitment to realise one's vision, and understanding why things are as they are, the practitioner can gain new insight into self and be empowered to respond more concretely in future situations within a reflexive spiral towards developing practical wisdom and realising one's vision as Praxis. The practitioner may require guidance to overcome resistance or to be empowered to act on understanding.' (Johns 2009, p.12)

> 'These emancipatory influences of critical theory are timely for contemporary nursing. If we want to educate and support critically responsive and sensitive practitioners, then reflection offers the potential for nurses to develop in their responsiveness and ability to take action in an often chaotic word of practice.' (Bulman and Schutz 2007).

Similarities and differences in explanations of reflection

You can probably appreciate by now that reflection is a difficult concept to explain. However, I hope you will notice some similarities; for instance, the exploration of experience, the analysis of feelings as well as oneself to inform learning. You will also see that many are influenced by critical theory where there is an assumption that reflection will involve a changed perspective and action. It is also possible to notice elements of experimentation and review, and purposeful learning through experience. There are inevitably differences too; not all emphasise the significance of feelings and emotion or explicitly recognise the inclusion of change, for instance. Additionally, some do not overtly mention the importance of having someone to reflect with, suggesting a more solitary interpretation of reflection.

Some key points about the concept of reflection

Essentially, reflection is more than simply being thoughtful (Jarvis 1992). What is clear is that the process of reflection has the potential to help nurses and other professionals to learn from their experiences. I have described it as reviewing experience from practice so that it may be described, analysed, evaluated, and consequently used to inform and change future practice in a positive way (Bulman 2008). I also believe that reflection involves opening up one's practice for others to examine, and consequently requires courage and open-mindedness, as well as a willingness to take on board, and act on, criticism (Dewey 1933). In addition, reflection involves more than 'intellectual thinking' since it is intermingled with practitioners' feelings and emotions, and acknowledges an interrelationship with action (Brockbank and McGill 1998). Ultimately and importantly, I would suggest that reflection in nursing is connected with a professional motivation to 'move on' and 'do better' within practice in order to learn from experience and critically examine 'self' (Bulman et al. 2012).

Noteworthy concepts for a deeper understanding of reflection

Praxis

You will have noticed that the quote by Johns (2009), describing reflection, mentions praxis. The concept of praxis originates from Greek philosophy and can be seen in the work of the educationalist and educational philosopher Paulo Friere, who has been influential in education throughout the world. He suggested that we need to reflect and act in the world in order to transform it and to develop our own critical awareness of it. Friere's (1972) notion of praxis or action that is informed and linked to certain values is significant to a deeper understanding of the concept of reflection. It is this notion of praxis that emphasises the requirement to make a positive difference to clients, to avoid 'automatic pilot' and strive to develop responsive and purposeful practice – to make a difference in the world. It may seem obvious, but this is important because people matter and we have a commitment to do the best that we can for our patients and families, in fact all those who need nursing. This emphasises the necessity for reflection to be more than just 'navel gazing' and reiterates the focus on improving practice.

Critical being

Friere's notion of praxis and the belief in its central place in any contemplation about reflection resonates with Barnett's (1997) notion of critical being. Principally, Barnett deconstructed the idea of traditional critical thinking within higher education. He advocated the nurturing of critical *being* in students rather than critical *thinking*. This moves away from concentrating on critical thinking as purely cognitive, or as something only done within the confines of higher education rather than in the 'real world' of practice. By its very nature, critical being encapsulates the development of critical thinking but also the critical development of self and a commitment to take action in the world. I would suggest that Barnett's notion of critical being has similarities with reflection as described above, because reflection involves an intermingling of different sorts of knowing that includes propositional knowledge, feelings, self-awareness and a commitment to action. Similarly to critical being, reflection is more than a cognitive process; it involves the cognitive plus the affective and active. Reflection does not do away with drawing on theory/research in order to make sense of a situation; it also values the importance of feelings as beneficial to rational thinking and the importance of change, development and action in order to learn from, and move on in, one's practice. Educational philosopher and feminist Nell Noddings (1984) captures the significance of the benefits of intermingling the rational and the emotional:

> 'If I exclude cognition, I fall into vapid or pathetic sentimentality; if I exclude affect – or recognise it only as an accompaniment of sorts – I risk falling into self-serving or unfeeling rationalisation.' (Noddings 1984, p.171)

In addition, Barnett eloquently expresses his vision for critical being:

> 'There has to be an attempt on the part of students seriously to come to know the world and to understand the self as a constituent of that world; there has to be a propensity to form an evaluation of both the world and the self; and there has to be a willingness to engage in the world so as to effect changes that are not purely instrumental. When all three exemplifications of the critical spirit are together – thought, action and self – we are in the presence of critical persons.' (Barnett 1997, p.87)

The key point is that it is this intermingling of the cognitive, affective and action through reflection that has the potential to help nurses make sense of practice and make a difference to it. Seen as a way of critical being, reflection becomes more than simply a technique that we can teach you (although it may feel like that at the outset!) but rather a way of being in practice and in life (Johns 2009). The interview extract below (Bulman 2009) illustrates this vision of reflection as a way of critical being:

'... I don't know if you remember when the Tiananmen Square massacre went on, but there was a bit of film of somebody with two bags standing in the middle of the road and a queue of tanks coming along and he was standing there. He wouldn't let them go past ... I believe we know who the person was now and I think they probably had bags full of papers and political pamphlets and what have you. But I was envisioning this person as somebody who had just come back from the supermarket, who was just on their way home to cook the tea and thought: I am not having these tanks coming down my road! So to stop them like that! But Barnett (in his book) uses that visual image to encapsulate the critical being. ... And so, you know, if ever I am stuck for an image to sum up what I am aspiring to and what I am aspiring for my students too, it is that guy standing in the middle of the road, because I think that is where you bring together what you think, what you feel, what you are, and you make your statement about the world or about clinical practice or about whatever it is.'

'Knowing more than we can tell'

As expressed in the research quote above, the ability to communicate practice is an essential part of being reflective. This connects with Polanyi's (1958) influential work offering a critique of objectivity as it was presented in science and philosophy in the mid 20th century. He suggested that complete objectivity, as attributed to science, is a false ideal, thus pointing out the requirement to look at how personal knowing influences and enhances the objective. He also argued for the need to appreciate the knowledge that is embodied through practical knowing, e.g. the nurse develops a 'feel' for what she does practically and bodily so that it becomes part of her knowing process. However, this kind of knowledge cannot always be articulated in words; therefore, in this sense, 'we know more than we can tell' (Polanyi 1967, p.4). This means that we will have knowledge that may never be expressed, but Polanyi (1958, 1967) still recommended seeking out ways to help people to communicate and express themselves as adequately as possible. What is exciting is that reflection can provide a means for doing just that.

The complexity and messiness of many practice issues can 'niggle away' at practitioners; this relates to Schön's (1983) description of the 'swampy lowlands' of practice problems and is something that you might recognise within your own practice experiences. The sorts of issues that bother nurses can be difficult and uncomfortable to express in words. Yet reflection can provide a route to give nurses the opportunity to find both their personal and professional voices. Indeed, both Clouder (2000) and Johns (2004) have considered the ability of reflection to develop professional voices that are able to challenge opposition and oppression in the workplace. Reflection can allow nurses to develop language through which they can ask questions about and communicate their nursing knowledge, and in doing so 'find their own voice'. This links back again with reflection being concerned with developing people who are able to challenge and question, in order to make a difference in the world.

However, being able to articulate a developing sense of critical awareness and doubt about the world of practice should also be viewed with an element of caution, especially in situations where nurses have a lack of ability or power to change things. This leads on to the last part of this section which introduces some ideas about the dangers of reflection.

The 'dangers' of reflection

I have returned to a paper by Stephen Brookfield (1993) who is a highly regarded educationalist and an expert in the field of critical thinking. His original paper was written for a nursing audience and highlights some of the issues we should be sensitive to in relation to reflective education. Whilst this work is a few years old now, I felt it needed reviving since it has some essential messages on developing critical thinkers that no-one has expressed as fluently as Brookfield and these should not be forgotten. Whilst Brookfield refers to critical thinking in his arguments, having listened to him speak at a reflective practice conference at Cambridge University in 2006, I feel that these interpretations very much apply to reflection. The data for his assertions were taken from critical incident responses by nurses, nurse educators and other healthcare providers and administrative personnel in workshops that Brookfield ran over several years.

He proposed that 'Impostership', 'Cultural Suicide', 'Lost Innocence', 'Road Running' and 'Community' are all issues that require particular consideration with regard to the development of critical thinkers. He described Impostership – presenting a public 'false self' (p.198) – as something commonly felt amongst practitioners, where imposters look and act like professionals in front of their students and peers, all the while knowing that they are putting on a show. Brookfield suggested that initially this presentation of a false self is done for reasons of survival, in order to demonstrate ourselves as competent practitioners to others. Yet it can also prevent us from becoming too complacent and confident by ensuring that we view our practice as being in constant change. However, he made the point that Impostership can also be destructive, particularly if we believe 'we are the only ones whose practice is uninformed and experimental and that we fall far short of the perfection we suspect is exemplified in our colleagues' (p.199). He highlighted that a feeling of Impostership inevitably accompanies experimentation and can actually be heightened by it. Eloquently, he recommended that:

'… it is important that we never lose the sense as professionals that we are often struggling in the dark, trying to draw meaning from contradictory and often opaque experiences. To feel this is to open up permanent possibilities for change and development in our practice.' (Brookfield 1993, p.201).

Brookfield also described how it is possible to commit Cultural Suicide through expressing our experiences of change and critical reflection, thus risking alienation from colleagues and organisational cultures. Through critical questioning of 'conventional assumptions and accepted proce-dures' (p.201), we can end up being excluded from a culture that formerly supported us. Thus nurses developing as reflective practitioners may be seen as 'subversive troublemakers', and the challenging of assumptions about practice issues may be seen almost as an act of betrayal. This sense of the alienation that can arise in developing a sense of critical awareness about practice resonated with my own research (Bulman 2009) and is illus-trated in the interview extract below. This practitioner had begun to develop the ability to question practice issues through her reflective edu-cation but expressed her growing sense of frustration as she looked at practice with different eyes:

'I think that working in isolation to do reflection and trying to move forward when you are part of the team is extremely difficult … If you are able to set up clinical supervision, then we would all be able to work to move forward and set aside time to actually reflect about the practice on the ward, and discuss individuals' difficulties … Working in isolation with reflection sometimes doesn't give you the benefits, because it causes frustration and you feel that you're constantly explaining to other people why you should do things in a certain way.'

In contrast to the potential for empowerment and transformation through the process of reflection, Brookfield has highlighted the notion of Lost Innocence. He described nurses' stories of critical reflection as having a quality of Lost Innocence, as they struggled to find the ultimate answers to their problems in practice. Brookfield expressed this as doomed to disappointment since:

'Lost innocence is the gradual realisation that the more clinical practice we put behind us, the more we become aware of its essentially inchoate nature, of the fact that learning nursing is an uninformed, unfinished project. We become progressively attuned to its complexity, its messiness, and its chaos, particularly when we are trying to put some purposeful experimentation into our practice.' (p.203)

So whilst we are adjusting to new, possibly empowering and liberating understandings of practice and of ourselves, Brookfield has warned us that we shouldn't forget that a sense of Lost Innocence may accompany reflection.

Brookfield suggested that the critical process can be slow, halting and incremental, as well as difficult, tiring work. He has vividly related this to the image of the coyote futilely chasing the far too agile, gravity defying Roadrunner bird off the edges of canyons and along a never-ending highway in the North American 'Roadrunner' cartoon.

'The moment when the coyote's realisation of his predicament causes his crash to the canyon floor has the same experiential quality as a particular moment in the rhythm of learning critical thinking. It is the moment when we realise that the old ways of thinking and acting no longer make sense for us, but that new ones have not yet formed to take their place.' (p.204)

So, whilst we might be open to change and challenge, such a state of limbo, Brookfield commented, is frighteningly uncertain, since as we abandon assumptions and meanings concerning practice that once supported us, this can have an effect on our confidence and we can crash 'to the floor of our emotional canyons, resolving never to go through this again' (p.204), until we go back for more because of the things that 'niggle away' at us about practice.

Finally, and perhaps more hopefully, Brookfield highlighted the importance of belonging to an emotionally sustaining, peer learning Community. By forming an appropriate peer network we can be reassured that our 'private anxieties are publicly experienced' (p.205). If we can share the common experience of reflection with colleagues, the sorts of insights that we can get from this experience can help us to cope with some of the dangers associated with reflection that Brookfield has outlined. This sharing of personal insights and experience can provide the motivation and commitment necessary in order to develop practice through reflection. The key message here is that the practice and education organisations and cultures that we work within can have a significant influence on supporting and challenging practitioners using reflection.

This echoes my research (Bulman 2009) in which postregistration students' discourses suggested that their working environments often promoted reflection because of the challenging nature of the practice setting, rather than one that was self-confirming, along with opportunities such as group reflection in practice settings. Students talked warmly about the benefits of being able to reflect with trusted and respected colleagues in practice:

'I find that if I keep thinking about things, like the person that I did for my assignment, I always make sure I go back to someone in our team – anywhere in the building, it doesn't matter for me – but I know I will go to someone who I know I can relate to and just talk things through, so that I do have some sort of cut-off point or some sort of resolution or … better understanding.'

Students mentioned questioning and discussing practice with colleagues when faced with difficult or challenging situations at work. This showed a commitment to teaching, facilitating, listening and being with colleagues and highlights the importance of a helpful environment for the development of reflective practice.

Evidence-based practice and reflection

I have included this section on evidence-based practice (EBP) because I believe that reflection can play an important part in the process. EBP is a fundamental component of modern healthcare in the UK and across the world. The importance of EBP for nursing has been very much influenced by the enormous amount of work that has been done within medicine supported by the Cochrane Collaboration. Sackett *et al.* (1996, p.71) have defined EBP for medicine as:

'… the conscientious, explicit, and judicious use of current best evidence in making decisions about the care of individual patients. The practice of evidence-based medicine means integrating individual clinical expertise with the best available external clinical evidence from systematic research.'

This highlights the motivation to apply the best available empirically gathered evidence to clinical decision making, so that we can judge whether treatments and interventions are effective. The logical and rational process of EBP is very much in evidence in current discourses about nursing practice and is part of the preparation and continuing education of modern professional nurses. The impetus behind this movement is clearly connected with improving quality of care and this is laudable. However, I would like to suggest that the teaching of EBP can all too readily overly concentrate on teaching skills for critiquing, synthesising and applying research to practice, without consideration of some of the other factors that Sackett and colleagues focus on as important for good practice. In the definition above, you will see that they mention 'clinical expertise'; this emphasises the importance of clinical 'know-how' and judgement in the process of EBP. They also consider the requirement to take into account the individual preferences and choices of patients as part of the process of EBP.

I would suggest that these two vital aspects of EBP can receive less attention in the education of nurses than the ability to search for, analyse and systematically apply research. Sackett *et al.* (1996, p.72) passionately suggested that: 'External clinical evidence can inform, but can never replace, individual clinical expertise, and it is this expertise that decides whether the external evidence applies to the individual patient at all and, if so, how it should be integrated into the clinical decision'. Consequently, it seems to me that we need to find ways to help our students and practitioners to develop their clinical judgement, and responses to individual patients, as well as their ability to apply empirical evidence. Reflection has the potential to provide this direction. This is because reflection can help nurses to develop their clinical judgement and explore their relationships with patients, particularly if this is facilitated through reflective dialogue with others, so that they can be both supported and challenged in the process. As a result, reflection offers the prospect of combining sensitivity with considerations of effectiveness, in partnership with patients, in a way that Sackett *et al.* suggest, but perhaps do not pursue.

McCarthy *et al.* (2010, p.103), in a book on values-based health and social care, have suggested that:

'A professional encounter with service users in health and social care settings is a unique situation which requires the professional to draw upon a vast range of knowledge and experience. The uniqueness of each encounter may be compared with the infinite varieties of patterns seen in a microscope view of snowflakes.'

They stressed that experiential learning is at the heart of improving clinical judgement and that connecting previous knowledge and experience in a discerning, thoughtful manner helps practitioners to develop expertise. Reflection has the capacity to do this and should be part of the process of EBP.

When there is a lack of empirical evidence, it is also important to draw on learning through experience, in order to inform clinical judgement. The example below illustrates that whilst as nurses we may be developing expertise in critically evaluating empirical evidence for practice, we should not forget to exercise our clinical judgement and our sensitivity in considering patients and their families. We should not lose sight of the things that we know through our practice.

Recently, I was preparing a session for my undergraduate nursing students looking at the use of touch in nursing and came across a review on the use and clinical effectiveness of touch as a nursing intervention by Gleeson and Timmins (2005). The paper provided a clearly conducted, objective literature review exploring the use and effectiveness of touch as a distinct aspect of nurse–patient communication. The authors carefully considered and logically determined that there was a lack of empirical evidence available, coming to the conclusion that the widespread adoption of touch as a caring intervention should be discouraged in the absence of research evidence and clear guidelines for practice. At this point, my heart sank.

First of all, I began to cynically consider why there was not enough evidence; lack of funding sprang to mind, as well as the problems of applying highly valued quantitative methodologies to this sensitive area of research. I felt frustrated that the authors had not considered how their findings related to their own experiences of practice and other embodied accounts in the literature (see Rombalski 2003); this lead to reflecting on my own years of practice experience. I recounted numerous occasions when I had used touch to communicate caring and compassion to my patients and their families – hands held on the long journey down to thea-tre, therapeutic back massages for a patient having to lie prone after a below-knee amputation, hugs for distraught family members whose rela-tives had just died, the many times I had held a hand in the night when patients couldn't sleep. I recollected how over the years I had taught my students about their privileged position as nurses and the need to care-fully contemplate the power and appropriateness of touch in order to show connection through caring. I remembered how I had learnt this through working with inspiring role models in practice. I even recalled what it was like to have the tables turned and be a terrified preoperative patient myself, soothed with a reassuring squeeze of my hand by an oper-ating department practitioner as I awaited surgery. I still believed in the importance of appropriate touch as part of compassionate nursing care, despite the fact that the evidence base was lacking.

My message is that we need to be critical about the process of evi-dence-based nursing and how it informs practice and develops nursing knowledge. Also, if evidence-based nursing is to be therapeutic to patients, it must involve thoughtful clinical judgement and the particular consideration of patients' needs. We must not forget that these are vital components of EBP. Reflection can provide the means by which we can investigate our clinical judgement and our connection with patients. As Nussbaum (1990) has suggested, real practical insight and understanding is a complex matter involving the whole soul, so much so that overtheoris-ing and not drawing on these can actually get in the way of vision.

Reflection for communicating practice knowledge

I want to expand on the notion of practical insight and understanding a little more and make the point that nursing knowledge is important and has a valuable contribution to make to healthcare. We need to find ways to articulate this professional knowledge to others in order to improve nursing practice, liberate learning about practice, and develop the potency of nursing voices (Johns 2009). Reflection offers the potential to do this. Ultimately, our motivation should be to find ways to deliver, and constructively consider, the care given to those in need of nursing. Whilst reflective education may not be the only way to question and challenge practice, it does provide a means by which nurses can critically express their practice, in a way that is viewed as valuable by them. It is true that nurses have always needed to learn from their experiences, since at the very least they are required to be safe to practise. Yet, reflection has the potential to develop criticality much further than this. This is because reflection can embody nurses within this knowing (communication about practice then becomes less sanitised; Morgan and Johns 2005), help nurses to directly relate their learning back into action, and give them a means by which they can articulate their practice knowledge (Bulman 2009).

Expressing oneself and one's practice requires a command of language, as well as a conducive working environment. This expression can be encouraged through facilitative dialogue with supervisors and mentors, the development of reflective writing and the judicious use of reflective frameworks (see Chapter 9 for more on this). Dunne (2007) has suggested that practitioners need not only a capacity to reflect but also the ability to articulate their practical wisdom or judgement in relation to practice. It is this, he claimed, that practitioners require since it concerns the improvement of practice. The language that can be developed through reflective education can provide a route to give nursing work more visibility, because it can enable nurses to find a way to express themselves and their practice.

The notion of 'voice' resonates particularly with the work of Belenky et al. (1997). Within their qualitative interview study, they explored women's ways of knowing, describing language as a tool for representing and communicating experience with others. Women talked of their 'voices' or 'points of view' being effectively silenced by oppressive forces in society, such as their education. (Belenky et al. did state that their work was not gender specific and so also applicable to men.) The key point here is that whilst nurses may have extensive practice repertoires, if they are not able to reflect on and communicate them, then this stays with them, undeveloped and unarticulated, and therefore does not challenge them, or others, or the organisations they work within.

Consequently, a reflective culture within nursing needs to be concerned with developing nurses' voices so that they can express their practice, consider and communicate its effects, and make a difference to it. Reflection, used in this way, has the potential to give more prominence to discourses about the everyday things that nurses do, since it gives more visibility to caring (Johns 2004). In nursing, these discourses may often be humanistic and concerned with caring for, and being with, people. This is about trying to make patients' journeys more bearable, as expressed through influential writing such as Campbell (1984) on the nurse as a skilled companion and Freshwater and Stickley (2004) on the importance of developing emotional intelligence in nurse education. It is a professional nursing discourse, which can be seen as different from an organisational one related to efficiency and cost-effectiveness. It also differs from a medical focus on symptom control and curing.

Given that there are these tensions between different discourses, all professionals need to find ways to communicate their discipline and professional knowledge to others. This is significant because nursing knowledge has the potential to make a positive difference to patients. From a broader perspective, communicating what nursing is about is vital for the development of the profession and ultimately for its survival as a discipline. This seems particularly important in the UK where presently we seem to be confronted with media that distrust the professionally educated nurse and where therapeutic and humanistic nursing care does not seem to be given the same value as productivity and meeting targets.

Empowerment and change

With reference to Friere's (1972) work, Jarvis and Gibson (1997) have commented that it might be assumed that all reflective learning must be revolutionary, but that reflective learning is not automatically innovative. In fact, nursing research has highlighted the powerlessness that nurses may have to change things (Paget 2001; Mantzoukas and Jasper 2004). In addition, in a meta-analysis of research and discussion papers on reflective practice, Gustafsson et al. (2007) highlighted that reflective practice appeared to be dependent on environment and context. They emphasised that such a constructivist movement, based on learning through experience, was overlooked in environments favouring scientific knowledge and management values. It is inevitable, then, that nurses struggle to find ways to express their practice. Thus practice informed by reflection can only take place where nursing work is not taken for granted and where the knowledge generated through reflection is seen as important.

Mantzoukas and Jasper's (2004) study of reflection has explored this difficulty. They suggested that the concept of reflection appears to be invalidated by the organisational hierarchy and power struggles in practice. For instance, in their study, it was ward nurses' perception that the types of knowledge they possessed were not as important as either the 'scientific' knowledge of doctors or the generalised, non-practice focused knowledge of management. In addition, reflection, as nurses attempted to use it, was viewed negatively by this dominant ward culture. Thus, as the researchers concluded, if the organisational culture disregards the nature of learning through reflection and does not support its use, then it is not likely to become evident in daily practice. All of this does serve to highlight the importance of the environment to change, if reflection is to be considered transformatory.

Yet, in terms of personal change, research does indicate nurses undergoing personal transformation and developing insights into the nature of nursing and of their practice (see Collington and Hunt 2006; O'Donovan

2007; Turner and Beddoes 2007). Equally there are other examples of nurses questioning and challenging their practice (Glaze 2001; Holmström and Rosenqvist 2004), as well as evidence that people felt that they had changed as individuals (Glaze 2001) and that they had continued to change after their formal education had finished (Paget 2001). This is reassuring since despite some of the dangers of reflection, there are some positive pay-offs. However, the crucial point is that practice environments seem to be just as essential to change as the focus on self-transformation. This requires grasping both the contextual and social issues to do with practice (Pryce 2002) if reflection is in any way to be emancipatory, i.e. people are able to act in a liberated way to change practice. In turn, for nurses to be empowered to change, it is evident that more than the courage and commitment of individuals is required, because although individuals seem to be changed by the process of reflection, the work environment plays a key role (Collington and Hunt 2006; O'Donovan 2007; Bulman 2009).

Nurse education and knowledge tensions

Nursing education in the UK has merged into higher education relatively recently, and this has had its tensions. It has meant existing within an education system that historically promotes the division of theoretical and practical knowledge and which traditionally denies an interrelationship between intellect and emotion (Brockbank and McGill 1998). This philosophical legacy promotes the idea that intellectual knowledge is different from, and superior to, practical knowledge. It originated from the early philosophers such as Plato, but was strongly influenced by later, popular Cartesian dualism which viewed the mind as something separate from the body. However, other philosophers began to appreciate thinking from a different stance. They argued that the mind and body are interconnected and that knowledge is socially rather than individually constructed, and therefore that thinking, feelings and action are intertwined (Ryle 1963, 1979; Wittgenstein 1967).

Eraut (1994) has emphasised the tensions between these university and professional perspectives on knowledge. Universities seek to develop and broaden academic knowledge and consequently to challenge long-established professional practices and thus these tensions may be viewed as beneficial. Yet, Eraut also discussed the difficulties with integrating professional education into higher education, citing the difference between propositional knowledge ('knowing that') and 'knowing how'. This is a point amply illustrated by the philosophers above, under the assumption that propositional knowledge is the most 'truthful' form of knowledge. This exposes the influence of western philosophy on the importance and status of propositional knowledge in western society and leads back to the old problem of dualism in the way that the nature of knowledge is appreciated.

Nurse education and reflection

A decade on from Eraut's (1994) observations, Meerabeau (2005) has expressed comparable tensions through her description of the 'inaudibility' of nursing within academia, and the oppression and disparagement that exist in attitudes towards practice knowledge and the expression of nurses' 'ideals of care'. Because of these sorts of tensions, nurses, along with other professionals, have been interested in reflection and consequently have contributed to the growing body of literature on the concept (Bulman et al. 2012). This is because reflection provides a way to communicate and justify the importance of practice and practice knowledge, as suggested by Johns (1995). This, in effect, would legitimise knowledge derived from the realities of practice rather than from more traditional forms of knowing (Brockbank and McGill 1998). Consequently, nursing education has been integrating reflection into the preparation and continuing professional development of nurses. In the UK, this can be specifically identified in recent Nursing and Midwifery Council publications (Nursing and Midwifery Council 2005, 2010).

Liberating and using practice experience

Nursing is a practice discipline and effective preparation of nurses should enable us to care competently for clients and continue to develop skills and knowledge over a professional lifetime. This means learning certain skills and particular knowledge, and developing attitudes and attributes that allow us to nurse in an effective and sensitive way that makes a positive difference to our clients (Paterson and Zderad 1988). A traditional way of achieving this is through what Schön (1987) called technical rationality, where students learn about theory and then apply this to their practice, thus separating intellectual and practical knowledge. No doubt many of you will be able to identify with this style of education when you look back at some of your own experiences.

I have expressed the lack of recognition of personal and practice knowledge in higher education generally and thus the issues for nurse education which now exists within it. In accordance with philosophical propositions about the nature of knowing, where thinking, feelings and action are intermingled (Ryle 1963; Wittgenstein 1967), it seems important for nurses to find ways to critically communicate their stories about practice in ways that cannot be achieved through a traditional technical route nor can be found in conventional nursing textbooks. The value of acknowledging and learning from this type of thinking and knowing is powerfully captured in Sue Duke's (2000, 2004, 2008) work on developing her reflection. The following small extract is typical of the sorts of stories that nurses tell about their everyday practice:

'Nursed a patient tired of fighting, feeling hopeless. I stayed with the patient but my heart emptied of anything that could protect me.' (Duke 2000, p.138)

What is significant is that after Sue wrote this extract, she began to reflect on it and described her astonishment in being able to capture her feelings about caring for this person. It was then that she began to speculate how many times she had felt like that before, yet had simply forgotten how she felt, and why. It began a long process of attending to, and reflectively writing about, her practice and gave her an opportunity to learn from it. You can read more of Sue's continuing journey in Chapter 7 of this edition.

Essentially, contemporary ideas about nursing advocate the need for nurses to be educated in ways that develop their autonomy, critical thinking, open-mindedness and ability to be sensitive to others (Freshwater and Stickley 2004). This reflects the demands and expectations made on today's nurses and the health services within which they work. In the nursing literature, reflection has been observed as a potentially useful strategy for developing these qualities in nurses and is a concept that is promoted in nursing education internationally (Ruth-Sahd 2003; Bulman and Schutz 2008; Freshwater et al. 2008). My own experiences of using reflection as well as with students and colleagues have also personally persuaded me of its value. In addition, Duke's example above illustrates the opportunity to liberate and use everyday practice experience, in order to learn from practice and explore its effects.

Conclusion

Getting prepared by reading about reflection, as you have just done, is a good start in getting an initial grasp of the concept and some of the current concerns connected with it. Through this introductory chapter, I have helped you to explore reflection, as well as encouraged you to regard it with a critical eye, and to consider it with regard to contemporary issues that affect nursing today. You have been able to consider different explanations of reflection and have been introduced to important concepts that help in a deeper appreciation of it, including praxis, critical being and tacit knowledge ('knowing more than we can tell'), plus some of the 'dangers' of reflection. I have also briefly considered the important role reflection can play in the EBP movement as a way of developing clinical judgement and sensitivity to clients and practice contexts. The chapter also guides you to consider key issues related to reflection, including communicating practice knowledge, empowerment and change, as well as knowledge tensions and the relevance of reflection in nurse education, before finally focusing on reflection as a way of liberating and using practice experience.

References

Atkins, S. and Murphy, C. (1993) Reflection: a review of the literature. *Journal of Advanced Nursing*, **18**(8), 1188–1192.

Barnett, R. (1997) *Higher Education: A Critical Business*. Society for Research into Higher Education/Open University Press, Buckingham.

Belenky, M.F., Clinchy, B.M., Goldberger, N.R. and Tarule, J.M. (1997) *Women's Ways of Knowing. The Development of Self, Voice and Mind*. Basic Books, New York.

Boud, D., Keogh, R. and Walker, D. (1985) *Reflection: Turning Learning into Experience*. Kogan Page, London.

Boyd, E.M. and Fales, A.W. (1983) Reflective learning: key to learning from experience. *Journal of Humanistic Psychology*, **23**(2), 99–117.

Brockbank, A. and McGill, I. (1998) *Facilitating Reflective Learning in Higher Education*. Society for Research in Higher Education/Open University Press, Buckingham.

Brookfield, S.D. (1987) *Developing Critical Thinkers. Challenging Adults to Explore Alternative Ways of Thinking*. Jossey-Bass, San Francisco.

Brookfield, S.D. (1993) On impostership, cultural suicide, and other dangers: how nurses learn critical thinking. *Journal of Continuing Education in Nursing*, **24**(5), 197–205.

Bulman, C. (2004) An introduction to reflection. In: Bulman, C. and Schutz, S. (eds) *Reflective Practice in Nursing. The Growth of the Professional Practitioner*, 3rd edn. Blackwell Scientific Publications, Oxford.

Bulman, C. (2008) An introduction to reflection. In: Bulman, C. and Schutz, S. (eds) *Reflective Practice in Nursing. The Growth of the Professional Practitioner*, 4th edn. Blackwell Scientific Publications, Oxford.

Bulman, C. (2009) Constructing reflection in nursing: a qualitative exploration of reflection through a post-registration palliative care programme. Unpublished PhD thesis. University of Southampton, School of Health Sciences.

Bulman, C. and Schutz, S. (2007) Practical wisdom in professional practice – contemplating some of the issues. Paper presented at Creating Phronesis, 13th International Reflective Practice Conference, June, Aalborg, Denmark.

Bulman, C. and Schutz, S. (2008) *Reflective Practice in Nursing*, 4th edn. Blackwell Scientific Publications, Oxford.

Bulman, C., Lathlean, J. and Gobbi, M. (2012) The concept of reflection in nursing: qualitative findings on student and teacher perspectives. *Nurse Education Today* **32**(5), e8–e13.

Campbell, A.V. (1984) *Moderated Love: A Theology of Professional Care*. Society for Promoting Christian Knowledge, London.

Clarke, D.J. and Graham, M. (1996) Reflective practice, the use of reflective diaries by experienced registered nurses. *Nursing Review*, **15**(1), 26–29.

Clouder, L. (2000) Reflective practice: realising its potential. *Physiotherapy*, **86**(10), 517–522.

Collington, V. and Hunt, S. (2006) Reflection in midwifery education and practice: an exploratory analysis. *Evidence Based Midwifery*, **4**(3), 76–82.

Dewey, J. (1933) *How We Think. A Restatement of the Relation of Reflective Thinking to the Educative Process*. DC Heath, Massachusetts.

Duke, S. (2000) The experience of becoming reflective In: Burns, S. and Bulman, C. (eds) *Reflective Practice in Nursing. The Growth of the Professional Practitioner*, 2nd edn. Blackwell Scientific Publications, Oxford.

Duke, S. (2004) When reflection becomes a cul de sac – strategies to find the focus and move on. In: Bulman, C. and Schutz, S. (eds) *Reflective Practice in Nursing. The Growth of the Professional Practitioner*, 3rd edn. Blackwell Scientific Publications, Oxford.

Duke, S. (2008) Continuing the journey with reflection. In: Bulman, C. and Schutz, S. (2008) *Reflective Practice in Nursing*, 4th edn. Blackwell Scientific Publications, Oxford.

Dunne, J. (2007) Practice and its informing knowledge: an Aristotelian understanding. In: Drummond, J.S. and Standish, P. (eds) *The Philosophy of Nurse Education*. Palgrave Macmillan, Basingstoke.

Eraut, M. (1994) *Developing Professional Knowledge and Competence*. Falmer Press, London.

Freshwater, D. and Stickley, T. (2004) The heart of the art: emotional intelligence in nurse education. *Nursing Inquiry*, **11**(2), 91–98.

Freshwater, D., Taylor, B. and Sherwood, G. (2008) *International Textbook of Reflective Practice in Nursing*. Blackwell Publishing, Oxford.

Friere, P. (1972) *Pedagogy of the Oppressed*. Herder and Herder, New York.

Glaze, J. (2001) Reflection as a transforming process: student advanced nurse practitioners experiences on developing reflective skills as part of an MSc programme. *Journal of Advanced Nursing*, **34**(5), 639–647.

Gleeson, M. and Timmins, F. (2005) A review of the use and clinical effectiveness of touch as a nursing intervention. *Clinical Effectiveness in Nursing*, **9**, 69–77.

Gustafsson, C., Asp, M. and Fagerberg, I. (2007) Reflective practice in nursing care: embedded assumptions in qualitative studies. *International Journal of Nursing Studies*, **13**, 151–160.

Habermas, J. (1977) *Knowledge and Human Interests*. Beacon Press, Boston.

Holmström, I. and Rosenqvist, U. (2004) Interventions to support reflection and learning: a qualitative study. *Learning in Health and Social Care*, **3**(4), 203–212.

Jarvis, P. (1992) Reflective practice and nursing. *Nurse Education Today*, **12**, 174–181.

Jarvis, P. and Gibson, S. (1997) *The Teacher Practitioner and Mentor in Nursing, Midwifery, Health Visiting and the Social Services*. Stanley Thornes Limited, London.

Johns, C. (1995) The value of reflective practice for nursing. *Journal of Clinical Nursing*, **4**, 23–30.

Johns, C. (2004) *Becoming a Reflective Practitioner*, 2nd edn. Blackwell Publishing, Oxford.

Johns, C. (2009) *Becoming a Reflective Practitioner*, 3rd edn. Wiley-Blackwell, Oxford.

Mantzoukas, S. and Jasper, M.A. (2004) Reflective practice and daily ward reality: a covert power game. *Journal of Clinical Nursing*, **13**, 913–924.

McCarthy, J., Alexander, P., Baldwin, M. and Woodhouse, J. (2010) Valuing professional judgement. In: McCarthy, J. and Rose, P. (eds) *Values-Based Health and Social Care: Beyond Evidence-Based Practice*. Sage Publications, London.

Meerabeau, L. (2005) The invisible (inaudible) woman: nursing in the English Academy. *Gender, Work and Organization*, **12**(2), 124–146.

Mezirow, J. (1981) A critical theory of adult learning and education. *Adult Education*, **32**(1), 3–24.

Morgan, R. and Johns, C. (2005) The beast and the star: resolving contradictions within everyday practice. In: Johns, C. and Freshwater, D. (eds) *Transforming Nursing Through Reflective Practice*. Blackwell Publishing, Oxford.

Mulhall, A. and Le May, A. (1999) Bridging the research–practice gap: a reflective account of research work. *Nursing Times Research*, **4**(2), 119–129.

Noddings, N. (1984) *Caring: A Feminine Approach to Ethics and Moral Education*. University of California Press, Berkeley, California.

Nursing and Midwifery Council (2005) *The PREP Handbook*. Nursing and Midwifery Council, London.

Nursing and Midwifery Council (2010) Standards for pre-registration education. http://standards.nmc-uk.org/PreRegNursing/statutory/background/Pages/more-standards-for-education.aspx

Nussbaum, M.C. (1990) *Love's Knowledge: Essays on Philosophy and Literature*. Oxford University Press, Oxford.

O'Donovan, M. (2007) Implementing reflection: insights from pre-registration mental health students. *Nurse Education Today*, **27**(6), 610–616.

Paget, T. (2001) Reflective practice and clinical outcomes: practitioners' views on how reflective practice has influenced their clinical practice. *Journal of Clinical Nursing*, **10**, 204–214.

Paterson, J.G. and Zderad, L.T. (1988) *Humanistic Nursing*. National League for Nursing, New York.

Polanyi, M. (1958) *Personal Knowledge*. Routledge and Keegan Paul, London.

Polanyi, M. (1967) *The Tacit Dimension*. Doubleday, New York.

Pryce, A. (2002) Refracting experience: reflection, post modernity and transformations. *Nursing Times Research*, **7**(4), 298–310.

Rombalski, J. (2003) A personal journey in understanding physical touch as a nursing intervention. *Journal of Holistic Nursing*, **21**(1), 73–80.

Ruth-Sahd, L.A. (2003) Reflective practice: a critical analysis of data-based studies and implications for nurse education. *Journal of Nursing Education*, **42** (11), 488–496.

Ryle, G. (1963) *The Concept of the Mind*. Penguin, Harmondsworth.

Ryle, G. (1979) *On Thinking*. Blackwell, Oxford.

Sackett, D.L, Rosenberg, W.M.C., Muir Gray, J.A., Haynes, B.R. and Richardson, S.W. (1996) Evidence based medicine: what it is and what it isn't. *British Medical Journal*, **312**, 71–72.

Schön, D.A. (1983) *The Reflective Practitioner*. Basic Books/Harper Collins, San Francisco.

Schön, D.A. (1987) *Educating the Reflective Practitioner*. Jossey-Bass, San Francisco.

Turner, D. and Beddoes, L. (2007) Using reflective methods to enhance learning: experiences of staff and students. *Nurse Education in Practice*, **7**(3), 135–140.

Van Manen, M. (1977) Linking ways of knowing with ways of being practical. *Curriculum Inquiry*, **6**(3), 205–228.

Wittgenstein, L. (1967) *Philosophical Investigations*. Blackwell, Oxford.

Wong, F.K.Y., Loke, A.Y.L., Wong, M., Tse, H., Kan, E. and Kember, D. (1997) An action research study into the development of nurses as reflective practitioners. *Journal of Nursing Education*, **36**(10), 476–481.

Chapter 1

Chapter 2

Developing skills for reflective practice

Sue Atkins[1] and Sue Schutz[1,2]

[1] Faculty of Health and Life Sciences, Oxford Brookes University, Oxford, UK
[2] University of Southampton, Southampton, UK

Introduction

This chapter is based upon our belief that there are certain skills underlying the development and use of reflective practice. We hope that you will find it useful. By now, if you have read about reflection and the potential it has for improving our practice, you may be wondering how you can become more skilled in using it. We present in this chapter some ideas that should help you to begin to develop the skills needed.

During the past 20 years, there has been much discussion and debate within nursing and healthcare literature about the nature of reflection and researchers have explored ways in which reflection can be facilitated in nursing courses (see Stewart and Richardson 2000; Glaze 2001, 2002; Hannigan 2001; Van Horn and Freed 2008). It is now widely understood that reflective practice is a process of learning and development through examining one's own practice, including experiences, thoughts, feelings, actions and knowledge. This means that reflection involves reviewing our own values, challenging our assumptions and considering the broader social, political and professional issues that are relevant to practice. These wider issues may be beyond our personal practice experience but are essential for us to consider if reflection is to result in significant and positive change. The skills that we need to achieve some of this change seem quite a 'tall order' and the aim of this chapter is to explore some of these and to give you some resources in order to develop them.

An early review of key literature on reflection from the fields of education and critical social theory suggested that the skills of self-awareness, description, critical analysis, synthesis and evaluation are necessary to engage in reflective practice (Atkins and Murphy 1993). More recent reviews by Duffy (2007), Mann *et al.* (2007) and Ruth-Sahd (2003) have

Reflective Practice in Nursing, Fifth Edition. Edited by Chris Bulman and Sue Schutz.
© 2013 John Wiley & Sons, Ltd. Published 2013 by John Wiley & Sons, Ltd.

added little to our understanding of the actual skills that we need in order to use reflection in our practice. Whilst current writers and researchers are pretty unanimous that reflection has potential, few give help and support to those who want to give it a try. In this chapter, we present a series of exercises that you can do that we believe will help.

We also offer an alternative perspective of developing reflective practice that may be useful for those of you who are more experienced practitioners. It is evident to us that the deliberate and systematic use of reflection as a learning tool in professional practice is a complex activity that needs to be consciously developed by pre- and post-qualifying professionals over time (Duke and Appleton 2000; Glaze 2001; Johns and Freshwater 2005). It is also more widely acknowledged that the development of reflection requires skilled, sensitive facilitation and appropriate guidance and support from educators, supervisors and mentors (Paget 2001; Brockbank and McGill 2007; Johns 2009). You will find that a variety of approaches are used to facilitate reflection. This includes the use of models and structured frameworks (see Chapter 9 for examples), reflective writing and journals (Bolton 2010), reflective dialogue (Brockbank and McGill 2007; Bolton 2010) and action learning sets (McGill and Beaty 2001). The intention of the skills-based approach, presented in this chapter, is to help you to use these tools more effectively.

A series of exercises is presented in this chapter, which are suggested for use by practitioners and facilitators, with a separate section devoted to each skill. The meaning of the skill is defined and explored, highlighting its relevance for both professional practice and academic work. The importance of each skill for reflective practice is justified with reference to key theories and recent research. The exercises enable you or your students to practise the skills of reflection alone, with a colleague or friend or within a group. We would recommend that you try both on-your-own and with-a-partner exercises because we believe that reflective dialogue and personal reflection are equally important.

The importance of underlying skills

An examination of the nature and process of reflective practice, as discussed by key and influential theorists, for example Mezirow (1981), Schön (1983) and Boud et al. (1985), suggests that there are underlying skills involved in reflective practice. The skills of self-awareness, description, critical analysis, synthesis and evaluation (Atkins and Murphy 1993) are implicit in the models and theories of these authors. For example, in Boud et al.'s (1985) analysis of the reflective process, the need to attend to our feelings and attitudes, in particular making use of positive feelings and dealing with negative feelings, is apparent throughout; this requires self-awareness. The stages labelled as 'Association', 'Integration', 'Validation' and 'Appropriation' involve varying degrees of critical analysis, synthesis and evaluation. Similarly, if we take Mezirow's (1981) concept of reflectivity and study its seven different dimensions, it is clear that self-awareness is integral at all levels The need for description, analysis, synthesis and evaluation becomes more evident when moving up the hierarchy from 'discriminant' to theoretical' reflectivity. Schön's (1983) analysis of the reflective practitioner's use of 'reflection-on-action' and 'reflection-in-action' implies the use of similar skills.

More recently, the development of structured models and frameworks to guide reflective practice in nursing and nurse education has made the use of these skills more explicit (Duke and Appleton 2000; Johns 2011). The importance of these underlying skills has been reinforced by a number of small-scale research projects that examine the development of reflection in students undertaking pre- and post-qualifying nursing courses. Jasper's (1999) study identified reflective writing as an important strategy for developing self-awareness and critical analysis. Duke and Appleton's (2000) study of palliative care students' development of reflective skills over an academic year demonstrated that reflective skills are acquired over time and that the higher level skills necessary for critical reflection are harder to develop and take longer to achieve. In Glaze's (2001) study of student advanced nurse practitioners' experiences of developing reflective skills, the practitioners describe their deepening self-awareness, greater critical analysis abilities (especially in relation to sociopolitical issues), and their efforts at synthesis and evaluation through attempts to empower colleagues and bring about changes in practice. You can see from these findings that skills are embedded in our understanding of what reflection involves.

You may have noticed from the last paragraph that there are similarities between the skills we need for reflective practice and the skills required for academic study. With the exception of self-awareness, these underlying skills are the higher order cognitive or thinking skills identified within Bloom et al.'s (1956) taxonomy of educational objectives. This taxonomy or hierarchy has guided and influenced the development of learning programmes, objectives and outcomes within higher education and you may have come across it if you have trained to be a mentor. Developing and refining these underlying skills may not only help us to develop a more reflective style of practice, but may further the development of our academic skills and our ability to integrate theory with practice. This is especially important for those undertaking work-based learning and professional development courses but is also vital for practice development.

Limitations of a skills-based approach to developing reflective practice

It is important to acknowledge the limitations of a skills-based approach to developing our reflection skills. As we have seen earlier, reflective skills are acquired and developed gradually through our practice over time, rather than 'done and dusted' in any one course or package. While these exercises involve reflecting on practice, frequently away from the clinical setting, it is important to acknowledge that reflective practice is a way of examining thoughts, feelings and actions while actually engaged in professional practice, as illustrated in Schön's (1983) work. We all have our individual styles of learning and may therefore learn better if we use techniques that suit us. Therefore, the extent to which each of us finds this skills-based approach helpful is likely to vary. Highly structured and gradually staged approaches to developing the skills for reflective practice may be more suitable for less experienced students on preregistration programmes, as indicated by the work of Burrows (1995). It has been suggested by Bolton (2010) that the use of structured frameworks and exercises may be restrictive and counterproductive to the development of creativity in professional practice. Bolton advocates a less structured, narrative approach in which practitioners write freely about their practice experiences and share their writing within a facilitated group. What is important is that you find out about all the different means available to you and select those that help.

In addition, we would like to say that other skills, not addressed in this chapter, are also important, especially when engaging in reflection with other people. These include skills of active listening, empathy, assertiveness, supporting and challenging and the planning and management of change (see Durgahee 1998; Page and Meerabeau 2000; Brockbank and McGill 2007). In particular, change management skills are important if the outcome of reflection is to have a positive impact on practice. It is recommended that you take a look at some of the literature on change management too.

An alternative approach to developing reflective practice

For more experienced practitioners, and for those of you who find a skills-based approach does not suit you, you could consider some of the work that has been undertaken to define an alternative approach to reflective practice. In our work, we have carefully considered the writing of Schön (1983, 1987) and have discerned some characteristics or attributes of more advanced reflective practice from his work. These open up the notion of the reflective practitioner rather more and view the concept of reflective practice as something that we can develop over time, possibly without taking educational courses but with a mentor or coach, whichever suits you best. Through participation in academic and practice-based courses, through reflection, supervision and through self-awareness, the experienced practitioner can develop these attributes. So, if you are already engaged in reflection and would like to enhance your skills further, or like the sound of this alternative approach we suggest that you turn to the section entitled 'Attributes of the reflective practitioner' at the end of this chapter.

Guidance on using the exercises in this chapter

In this chapter, three types of exercises are presented.

- *On-your-own exercises*. You can undertake these alone, without a facilitator. It is recommended that about 15–30 minutes be spent on each of these exercises.
- *With-a-partner exercises*. These you should try with a colleague or fellow student. These exercises will take approximately 30–60 minutes.
- *With-a-group exercises*. These are to be undertaken in a group with a facilitator. These exercises will take between 30–90 minutes.

All exercises require a commitment of time and thought, just as reflection does. Taking the exercises slowly over several weeks is recommended as the best approach. It will also be helpful to refer to the many examples and extracts of reflection within other chapters of this book.

Issues for facilitators

It is recommended that facilitators of reflection be educators or supervisors who are experienced and feel comfortable working with adult learners. Those of you who are facilitators are reminded of the importance of role modelling and that you need to be a reflective practitioner or reflective teacher yourself. There is a wealth of literature focusing on the development of the reflective teacher and the facilitation of reflective learning, including, for example, Light and Cox (2009), Driscoll (2007), Brockbank and McGill (2007), Scanlan and Chernomas (1997) and Brookfield (1995).

As a facilitator, we would strongly recommend that you prepare carefully for a session facilitating reflection. Here are some top tips.

- Review all the exercises that you are asking the group to undertake from a personal point of view, as well as from an educational perspective. If you have not had the opportunity to engage in the exercises as a participant prior to being a facilitator, it is recommended that you at least challenge yourself with the on-your-own exercises.
- Be prepared to role model, or participate, in all exercises. It is essential that you as the facilitator demonstrate an openness and willingness to share experiences. After all, this is what you are asking the group to do. Some participants may see reflecting on experiences as uncomfortable and challenging. Facilitators can provide support and encouragement by example.

- Co-facilitation is suggested, depending upon the size of the group. With more than one facilitator, participants can benefit from the increased accessibility of a facilitator. The facilitators may also benefit from arranging to engage in ongoing dialogue and reflection with a peer.
- Bearing in mind the limitations of such a programme of exercises, and the fact that they are in no way intended to be comprehensive, facilitators should be prepared to guide participants to further appropriate resources.
- Ground rules need to be established when working with a group in this way. These might include agreement about listening to each other with respect, giving and being open to support, time management and keeping confidences. In our experience, these are potential pitfalls.
- Consider taking advantage of information technology where appropriate. E-learning and electronic discussion boards in particular are really useful ways to get students from disparate geographical areas reflecting together.

Self-awareness

To be self-aware is to be conscious of our character, including beliefs, values, qualities, strengths and limitations. It also encompasses the social self – this is developed through the way that others influence and shape us, including our culture, educational experiences and how we have experienced our socialisation. Burnard (1997) distinguishes between the inner self, how we feel inside, and the outer self, the aspects of us that other people see, including our appearance and our verbal and non-verbal behaviour. Self-awareness may be described as the foundation skill upon which reflective practice is built. It underpins the entire process of reflection because it enables us to see ourselves in a particular situation and honestly observe how we have influenced it and how the situation has affected us. Self-awareness enables us to analyse our own feelings, beliefs and values, as part of the social world, and is an essential part of the reflective process.

It is evident from some of the most influential literature that it is the use of self-awareness and personal knowledge which differentiates reflective learning from other types of mental activity, for example logical thinking and problem solving (Mezirow 1981; Boud et al. 1985). Indeed, all adult learners need to be self-aware in order to take responsibility for identifying and responding to their own learning needs and to consider how this affects others. It is also important, although obvious, to state that self-awareness is essential not only for reflective learning but for skilled professional nursing practice. In particular, knowledge of our own beliefs, values and behaviour and how these affect others is essential for developing good interpersonal skills and building therapeutic relationships with patients. In some ways, self-awareness is hard to avoid, as self-interest is part of human nature. However, developing an honest self-awareness is more complex. It is natural to want to see and portray ourselves in the most favourable light. This desire, together with our own prejudices and assumptions, can sometimes interfere with the ability to take a more objective look at ourselves. Therefore, being honest about who we really are requires courage, confidence, a certain degree of maturity and the support of others.

In particular, to develop and maintain an appropriate level of self-awareness in the work situation, and for reflective practice, requires substantial effort and mental energy. In nursing, we are sometimes dealing with deeply held values and strong feelings which may be uncomfortable and anxiety provoking. There may, therefore, be times when we choose to avoid the process and when it becomes more appropriate just to go home and relax. However, it is important to bear in mind that identifying and releasing our feelings, both positive and negative, is generally better for us, provided that the time and place are appropriate. Whilst a degree of personal insight and self-awareness is necessary to engage in reflective practice, it is also important to recognise that too much negative introspection and analysis can have an adverse effect. Therefore, there is a need to gain the right balance in any situation.

The following series of exercises aim to help you to identify and clarify your own beliefs, values and feelings. There are also exercises enabling you to examine your motivation for developing a more reflective type of practice, and the degree to which you are open and receptive to new ideas. These factors have been identified as essential prerequisites for reflective practice (Boud *et al.* 1985; Wong *et al.* 1997).

On-your-own exercise: **Clarifying values**
(15 minutes)

A personal value can be described by a statement that says what is important and significant to you as an individual in either or both of your professional and personal lives. Describe three of your own values below by completing this sentence:

It is important to me that:

1. ....
2. ....
3. ....

With-a-partner exercise: **Exploring values**
(30 minutes)

- Are you both clear and certain about what your values are? Give examples. Identify together some values that are key for you both.
- Do your values always guide your actions? Give examples of when they have done and when they have not.
- How did you acquire the key values in your life? Identify specific people or situations that have affected your values.
- Compare your answers and consider how you can become clearer about your own values.

Values perform an important function for everyone. They provide a clear framework for our perspectives on life and they provide a basis for our actions. Being clear about your values in professional practice is also important because it will help you to live with the results of your actions. What is interesting about values is that they are chosen but they are not necessarily consistent with one another; often, we come across situations in practice where our values conflict. For this reason, it is important to be clear about our motivations.

 On-your-own exercise: **How motivated am I?**
(15 minutes)

Think about the reasons why you want to develop the skills to use reflection. Make a list of these.

You may have identified some good reasons for becoming a reflective practitioner. In addition to enabling you to develop and enhance your nursing practice, reflection is important within formal professional courses, when profiling learning for professional registration purposes, for the assessment and accreditation of prior experiential learning (APEL) and for demonstrating work-based learning. If, however, you believe you have little to gain personally or professionally, you may find it more difficult to devote the necessary time to developing the skills you will need. There is always the possibility that this is not the right approach for you or that this is not the right time for you to undertake the exercises.

If you are working on these exercises alone, try teaming up with a colleague who is willing to try them out too – this may help to get you motivated.

> ⚇ *On-your-own exercise:* Am I open to new ideas?
> *(30 minutes)*
>
> Identify from your professional practice a situation where a colleague
> introduced a change that would or did have implications for your own
> practice.
>
> - Describe what the change was.
> - What were the significant background factors to this change?
> - What were your thoughts about it?
> - Identify your feelings about the change.
> - How receptive were you to the change? Why was this?
> - What were the prejudices and biases that influenced your
>   receptiveness?

This exercise may have highlighted two issues. First, change may not
necessarily be for the better. It may be that you have had negative feelings towards a change and that this was because you did not see the
change as being in the best interests of the team or the patients. It may
be that you felt that there was insufficient evidence to support the change.
Second, you may find change in itself difficult; if so, you need to consider
carefully the reasons why you feel this way. Changes can make us feel
insecure and unsettled. There may also be some periods in your life when
you are more receptive to change than at other times. However, it is
important to remember that openness to new ideas is necessary to be a
reflective practitioner. Working through some of the exercises will help
you to develop a more positive approach to change; it can be uncomfortable and a good facilitator or supportive colleague can help.

> ⚇ *On-your-own exercise:* Your life map
> *(15–30 minutes)*
>
> On a large piece of paper, draw a map or diagram that represents the
> background and history of your nursing practice or training. Include as
> much detail as possible. Putting your nursing practice into a picture
> format may seem awkward or difficult at first, but it will allow you to
> see your career from a very different perspective. Don't worry about
> drawing things correctly, just try to be creative.
>   Include as many of the following events as possible.
>
> - Your starting point
> - Achievements
>
> *Contd.*

- Joys
- Sadnesses
- Important people
- Obstacles

 With-a-partner exercise: **Directions and destinations** *(30–60 minutes)*

Take turns explaining the map of your career in nursing or in training. Give as much detail as possible, so that your partner can understand your background.

When listening to your partner, pay close attention to the details. Ask questions to better understand your partner's experiences. Also, listen for what is left out of your partner's story. Here are some questions you may want to use to probe a little deeper.

- Where are you on your map? How active or passive are you?
- Where are the strongest emotions on your map? What are these emotions? Have any emotionally strong experiences been left out?
- Are there any other people on your map? Who are they? Is anyone missing who should be there?
- Are there patients on your map? Why or why not?
- What takes up the most space on your map? Why do you think it does?
- Are there any empty spaces on your map? Should something else be included in those spaces? Is there any meaning in the emptiness?

 Group exercise: **Looking for the crossroads** *(30–60 minutes)*

All participants should post their 'maps' on the walls of the room. Without describing or analysing the maps, look for what is common.

- Themes
- Symbols
- Depictions
- Colour choices
- Any developments or sequences (e.g. from left to right, bottom to top)

Given the fact that members of a reflective practice group have lived through similar times and are engaged in the same profession, it isn't surprising that there may be common areas. Consider how you can value the shared experiences since they can bind a group or team together and can also provide support. Also, look for the differences between the 'maps'. These unique versions are valuable to the group in a different way in providing new perspectives. Spend a few minutes talking about the experience of 'mapping.' Allow each participant a chance to answer the question:

- What was the biggest surprise or insight you got from your own or others' life maps?

Doing life maps reminds us of the positive aspects of our careers, but it will also bring to mind the low points or sadnesses that we have experienced. Group members and facilitators should be prepared to support members of the group who need it.

Description

To describe something, whether it is a person, an object, a situation or an abstract concept or idea, is to state its characteristics or appearance without expressing a judgement. A descriptive account is usually in spoken or written form, but may also be in other forms, such as a painting or sculpture.

In appreciating the qualities and power of good description, examples of excellent descriptive accounts are widely available within English literature. In particular, we would refer you to Styles and Moccia's (1993) anthology entitled *On Nursing: A Literary Celebration* which contains many rich descriptive accounts of nursing, and people's experiences of health and illness. Outside nursing, the many novels of Charles Dickens contain superlative description and may provide you with an entertaining break from the nursing literature.

In professional practice, good descriptive abilities are necessary when we are communicating verbally with our colleagues about patients and when we are writing clear and accurate patient progress notes. When using reflection, description is the skill with which you recollect the important events and features of a situation or event. Good description is about giving a clear and comprehensive account of a situation. Your account should include the following key elements.

- Significant background factors (the context)
- The events as they unfolded in the situation,
- What you were thinking at the time

- How you were feeling at the time
- The outcome of the situation

Your description should reconstruct the situation, to enable someone who was not there to understand the situation from your position. What you are trying to do is paint a vivid picture that then allows you and others to review the situation.

Some people are gifted with the skill of description while others struggle to find the most appropriate words to express themselves. A full vocabulary is necessary to be able to describe situations but at the same time, there is a need to avoid jargon and terminology which the reader or listener may not understand. It is also important to discriminate between relevant and irrelevant information. A good descriptive account, therefore, demonstrates a full and clear understanding of the relevant and important issues, and is well structured and concise.

Within a piece of written reflection, or when engaging in reflection with another person or a group, it is also important that you achieve a balance between description of the situation and of the analytical processes which follow. In particular, when we are undertaking work for academic purposes, it is often the higher order thinking skills of analysis and evaluation that are most valued by our teachers. However, it may be more difficult to engage in these critical thinking processes without good underlying descriptive skills.

On-your-own exercise: The power of description (30 minutes)

Choose a page of literature from a favourite text, for example a novel, autobiography or poem. Read it carefully. When you feel that you are really familiar with the passage, write down:

- key elements of the description which capture the essence of the situation.
- important words or phrases which facilitated your understanding.

It is important to consider what the elements of good description are. If you are able to incorporate these into your writing, you are more likely to give the comprehensive account that enables you to demonstrate your learning through experience. A good piece of description paints a vivid picture of a unique situation. It enables the reader to understand the situation from the writer's perspective. The description contains details that not only capture the significant background factors but also bring to life the situation through the use of carefully selected words.

On-your-own exercise: 'I remember when ...'
(30 minutes)

Identify a work situation in which you were involved recently. The situation might include one or more of the following features.

- You felt that your actions made a real difference to a patient or group of patients.
- It went unusually well.
- It did not go as planned.
- It was very ordinary and typical of your professional practice.
- It captures the essence of what your professional practice is about.

Take some time to think about the situation. Bearing in mind the features of good description, write down as many of the details that you can remember. You need to avoid using the specific names of people or places involved, to preserve anonymity and confidentiality. Be sure to include information on the following.

- Where and when the situation occurred.
- Who was involved in the situation.
- The specific circumstances of the care provided/not provided.
- How you felt about the situation at the time.
- What you did at the time of the situation.
- How you coped after the situation.
- What you thought and felt about the situation at a later time.

With-a-partner exercise: 'Let me tell you about ...'
(30–60 minutes)

Using your notes from the on-your-own exercise, take it in turns to tell your partner of your experience. Don't be limited by what you wrote. Use your notes as a starting point. When listening to your partner, pay close attention to the details. Ask questions to better understand your partner's experiences. Also, listen for what is left out of your partner's story. You may want to probe a little deeper. In telling this story, did you talk more about what you felt, thought and did, or did you describe the actions and attitudes of others?

To facilitate another person's understanding of a situation, you need to give all the relevant factors in enough detail. A common problem may be that because you were involved in the situation, you may omit certain details that you have taken for granted. You may also find it difficult to recall all the key factors in the situation because you have to rely on your memory. It is likely that the situations you will be most easily able to describe are those that occurred more recently. Sometimes it is necessary to describe situations from your nursing practice that occurred some time ago. Keeping a diary that records and describes events in your professional practice may therefore enhance your descriptive abilities and also help you to work out what are the essential features (see Chapter 3 for more on diary keeping).

On-your-own exercise: Describing feelings (30 minutes)

Think of a situation in your professional practice where the outcomes were not what you expected or you felt uncomfortable about them. Describe the situation using the elements of good description, and then answer the following questions.

- Does your description capture the essence of the situation?
- Does what you have written describe your feelings accurately and truthfully?

It is not always easy to describe the feelings you have. Some of us find it easier to describe our thoughts about a situation rather than our feelings. When feelings are strong, for example when we are very happy or very upset, feelings tend to be easier to acknowledge. However, in any situation there are likely to be feelings beneath the surface that may need more detailed exploration to uncover. Some people find it easier to express feelings than others. If this is true for you, you need to consider some of the reasons why this might be the case. However, it is generally believed that we are better off identifying and releasing feelings (Boyd and Fales 1983; Brockbank and McGill 2007).

Critical analysis

Critical analysis is also a key skill for both reflective practice and academic study. Analysis involves the separation of a whole into its component parts. To analyse something, whether an object, a set of ideas or a situation, is to undertake a detailed examination of the structure or constituent parts or elements and ask questions about them, in order to more fully understand their nature and how the parts relate to, and influence, each other. The term 'critical' introduces a further dimension to analysis, in that judgements are made about the strengths and weaknesses of the different parts, as well as of the whole. Being critical does have some negative connotations when it is used in everyday life, as it is a term often associated with finding fault. However, engaging in critical analysis, or undertaking a critique of something, is a positive and constructive process, because it is about identifying strengths as well as weaknesses. Weaknesses can be seen more helpfully as opportunities for change and to move on. Examples of using critical analysis in professional practice include assessing the needs of an individual patient, as well as making a broader contribution to service and policy development.

Some authors emphasise critical analysis as a rational, linear, problem-solving process grounded in the scientific approach (e.g. Fisher 1995). However, the more widely accepted view appears to be that critical analysis and critical thinking involve an emotional dimension (Brookfield 1991; Daly 1998; Light and Cox 2009). Acknowledging and analysing beliefs, values and feelings are a fundamental and important part of reflection if the outcome is to have a positive effect on our professional learning, practice and ultimately the quality of patient care. As a healthcare professional, the situations you are involved in may be unique and therefore the knowledge that you need in order to understand and solve problems in practice will depend upon the individual components of the situation and the broader context. It is also important to recognise that any situation will be influenced by your own feelings, attitudes and behaviour. When engaging in reflective practice, therefore, the skill of critical analysis involves the following activities.

- Identifying and illuminating your existing knowledge that is relevant to the situation.
- Exploring your feelings about the situation and the influence that these have.
- Identifying and challenging any assumptions you may have made.
- Imagining and exploring alternative courses of action (Brookfield 1987).

Identifying your existing knowledge

The knowledge that you need to understand what is happening in a specific situation needs to be identified and scrutinised. You may find that in order to shed light on that situation, you need to search for, and examine, knowledge that at first may not have seemed relevant. It is therefore important that you identify the types and sources of knowledge that you use in your professional nursing practice. This is about raising questions such as: ' What do we know?' and 'How do we know it?'.

Professional knowledge, and nursing knowledge in particular, has been classified in a number of different ways (Carper 1978, 1992; Higgs and Titchen 2000). While recognising that any classification is artificial and that different types of knowledge are interdependent, it is sometimes helpful to refer to a framework or classification when examining our own knowledge. In western philosophy, a common distinction is made between propositional knowledge, or 'knowing that' (this comprises our theoretical knowledge and knowledge generated through research), and non-propositional knowledge, or 'knowing how'(which consists of our personal knowledge, our practical skills, our informal knowledge and expertise) (Polanyi 1958; Higgs and Titchen 2000). The work of Carper (1978, 1992) has been influential within nursing theory and is used in some frameworks for reflection, for example Johns (2011).

Carper identifies four fundamental patterns of knowing from an analysis of the structure of nursing knowledge.

- *Empirical knowledge* – factual, descriptive and theoretical knowledge, often developed through research.
- *Aesthetic knowledge* – knowledge gained more subjectively, through unique and particular situations, sometimes referred to as the art of nursing.
- *Personal knowledge* – knowledge of self, used for example in building therapeutic relationships with patients and in helping them cope with illness.
- *Ethical knowledge* – concerned with understandings and judgements of what is right, wrong or ought to be done in different situations.

So, if we consider Carper's ideas here, it is clear that engaging in a thorough critical analysis involves analysing our knowledge and, where necessary, actively seeking out the ideas, theories and research of others in order to look at them critically in the light of what we personally understand.

Exploring feelings related to the situation

In reflective practice, it is necessary to gain an appropriate balance between the analysis of knowledge and the analysis of feelings. It is also important to focus on our positive feelings as well as trying to deal with our negative feelings, in order for the process to be constructive (Boud *et al.* 1985). Not only are we concerned about how our feelings affect the care we give, but to be reflective, we must also be aware of, and constructively use, our own emotions.

Identifying and challenging assumptions

Identifying our assumptions is about recognising when we take something for granted or accept what others present as fact without other supporting evidence. It is about not taking things at face value but is about developing a critical approach. When analysing a situation, it may be helpful to ask questions like: 'What is being taken for granted here?'

and 'Am I representing an accurate picture of the situation?'. It may be easy to carry on through our working and personal lives with the same set of assumptions, beliefs and values about ourselves, about nursing and about healthcare practice in general. However, there is a need for us to challenge these assumptions regularly and to question where they have come from. Indeed, Jarvis (1992) suggests that we can easily miss crucial factors in practice by not seeing 'the extraordinary within the ordinary'; we have to see the situations that we take for granted in a different way. Challenging the relevance of the context of our nursing practice is particularly important. Events are embedded within a certain context, so it is important to be able to examine the ideas of people from different backgrounds, alongside our own. Assuming that ideas and practices that work in one context can automatically be carried to another can cause problems. Examples of such difficulties have sometimes been evident in attempts to apply North American nursing models and healthcare systems to nursing in the UK.

When we are identifying and challenging our assumptions, it is important for us to be sceptical of any claims to universal truth. The fact that a practice has existed for a long time does not mean that it is the most appropriate. Just because an idea is accepted by others does not mean that we have to believe in its innate truth, without first checking its correspondence with our own experience (Brookfield 1991). Challenging the assumptions underlying our own ideas and those of others can be an uncomfortable experience and may involve asking awkward questions. It is therefore important to raise our own awareness and to prompt, nurture and encourage the process in others without making them feel threatened.

Imagining and exploring alternative courses of action

Central to this is the notion of constantly looking for new ways of thinking and new ways of doing things. Such new ways of practising allow for creativity and growth as opposed to routine and stasis. You could ask yourself the following questions: 'Do I still work in the same way as I did two years ago? Is that appropriate? What, if anything, do I want to do about that?'. This aspect of critical analysis also requires us to look at perspectives other than our own.

 On-your-own exercise: Analysing your knowledge (30 minutes)

Take a situation previously described. Think about the knowledge that has enabled you to understand the situation. Write a detailed account of relevant knowledge and indicate the sources of the knowledge.

Some of the knowledge you have used is likely to have been gained through personal experience. Remember that while this is a useful and valid way of gaining knowledge, you need to explore the extent to which this knowledge helps you understand the situation. Some knowledge may have been gained through 'trial and error'. It is particularly important to question this knowledge and its value just as we would with any form of understanding. Evidence-based professional practice demands that formal knowledge must be a key source of understanding and it is important that your understanding of any situation includes research-based knowledge where appropriate. If you have been unable to identify any formal sources of knowledge, it may be that you need to do some further thinking and reading. Cultural knowledge contained within groups such as nursing teams can be more difficult to identify, as this knowledge is often implicit in everyday practice. It may be taken for granted or be bound up in the assumptions that underlie your practice. It is important that you explore any assumptions you may make.

 With-a-partner exercise: Discussing your knowledge (30–60 minutes)

Ask a partner to read the situation you described previously. Discuss together the knowledge which each of you considers is relevant to understanding the situation.

- Was the knowledge that your partner identified the same as or different from yours?
- If different, explore the reasons why.
- Agree with your partner which type of knowledge is most important for understanding the situation.
- Try to identify together any new knowledge that would be relevant to the situation, and suggest alternative knowledge which may give new insights.

 On-your-own exercise: Analysing your feelings (30 minutes)

Taking a situation described previously, identify any parts that involved feelings. Read through the section carefully. See whether you have identified your feelings where appropriate. If not, why not? Try to explore honestly why you felt the way you did.

If necessary, try again to identify your feelings. Taking the relevant passage, think carefully and identify the feelings that were important in that situation. This may include feelings you had within the situation and about it, the feelings you had at the time and the feelings you have now.

Contd.

Answer the following questions.

- Why did you feel the way you did?
- What are the elements that made you feel that way?
- Was there anything relevant in your past experiences which led you to feel the way you did?

 With-a-partner exercise: Talking about feelings (*30 minutes*)

Talk through your feelings with someone you trust.

Reflective practice always involves an analysis of our feelings and without this understanding, you may miss real opportunities to learn about yourself. Increasing self-awareness and the ability to analyse your feelings will give you insights that may enhance your professional practice. While analysis of feelings is difficult, if you have not been able to undertake this exercise, you need to consider carefully the reasons why.

 On-your-own exercise: 'One way of looking at it' (*30 minutes*)

Critically analyse a situation previously described, from as many different perspectives as possible. Try to imagine the point of view of patients, colleagues and other people who were involved in the situation.

 With-a-partner exercise: 'Different ways of looking at it' (*30–60 minutes*)

Practise taking opposing opinions on the situation presented in the previous exercise. Try defending a perspective that is not your own. Support your views with formal knowledge or theory where possible.

Frequently, healthcare professionals operate from substantially different viewpoints. When a dilemma presents itself, people react differently based on their beliefs and experience. The resulting conflict can be both upsetting and baffling. It may be hard sometimes to understand how equally concerned caregivers can have opposing opinions. However, in a climate of interprofessional working it is becoming increasingly important to understand and respect the values of others. Do not overlook the richness of diversity. We are open to differences in our patients and clients and need to be equally open to differences in our own professional relationships.

 Group exercise: The great debate
(30–90 minutes)

Divide the group into several teams, depending on the size of the group. Each team should identify and will then represent a key theory used in professional nursing practice. The teams should be asked to debate the following question.

• What theory provides the most value to healthcare providers?

Team members should work together to develop their arguments. One or two members of the team should be selected as spokespersons for the group.

Round 1 – each team is allowed 5 minutes to state why their theory is the most useful to healthcare providers.
Round 2 – each team is given 5 minutes to state the reasons why the other theories presented are inadequate in meeting the needs of healthcare providers.

Success of the teams will be based on the clarity of their communication and arguments.

Synthesis

Synthesis is defined in the *Oxford Dictionary* as 'the process or result of building up separate elements, especially ideas, into a connected and coherent whole'. It could be described as the opposite of analysis. Synthesis is about the artistry of our professional practice and about being creative. It often involves original thinking about novel solutions. At a fundamental level of practice, devising a patient care plan is an example of the synthesis of information from a variety of different sources. A good care plan is unique to the individual patient and is dynamic and changing.

When using reflection, synthesis is the ability that you need to integrate new knowledge, feelings or attitudes with your previous knowledge, feelings or attitudes. This is necessary in order to develop a fresh insight or a new perspective on a situation and therefore to learn from it. Therefore, the skill of synthesis is necessary in order to achieve a satisfactory outcome from reflection. This may include the clarification of an issue, the development of a new attitude or way of thinking about something, the resolution of a problem, a decision made or a change in behaviour. Such changes may be small or large. New knowledge may potentially be generated and original ideas or fresh ways of approaching problems or answering questions may be developed. Synthesis involves us making choices with regard to relating new ideas to our past beliefs and values. This may not be an easy process, depending upon the scope of adjustment that you have to make. You may choose not to incorporate new ideas and instead maintain the existing ones; this is not necessarily right or wrong. Changing old ideas should not be done indiscriminately. The important point is that the choice is an informed decision.

The skill of synthesis can be a difficult one. Listening to the way others have put the pieces together in relation to different situations may be helpful at this point.

 On-your-own exercise: **'Dear friend ...'**
(30 minutes)

Take some time to think about what you have learned from the previous exercises and write a letter to a friend, real or imagined, telling of the changes you have experienced. Be sure to include some of the following.

- Give an update on yourself and your self-awareness. Has it changed? What did you learn by mapping out your career and talking it over with a partner?
- Describe one of the situations that you believe has most influenced your practice.
- Include information about the knowledge or theory you believe has most relevance to your practice.
- Finish off by writing about what you intend to do differently in identifying and handling some of the issues you encounter in your practice.

With-a-partner exercise: **Spotlight on you**
(30–60 minutes)

In addition to the written reflections that you have undertaken during these exercises, you now have the opportunity to make an audio-visual recording. By recording your thoughts, you will be able to hear and see yourself express your views about your nursing practice. You will also

Contd.

be able to use the recording as a yardstick against which to measure your professional growth in the future. On completion, the record will be yours alone. There will be no need to share it with anyone other than your partner for the exercises. However, you may choose to show it to a facilitator, friend, family member or mentor, or you may decide to view it again in the privacy of your own home. You have done all the preparation for this experience in the previous exercises. There is no need to use notes or check your readings. Your partner will prompt you with the questions listed below.

1. Tell me a little bit about who you are. (Remember the information you put in the map of your career. You may wish to add to that information.)
2. Think of a meaningful incident in your professional career. Tell me:

- what your role was
- what were the choices you had to make
- what the choice you made was
- how you felt about your choice.

You do not need to use the incident you described previously in the section on description. Discussion of that incident may have brought to mind other situations that you have faced in practice.

3. What type of work would you like to see yourself ultimately doing? What changes and improvements would you make in the way you approach and handle the issues that you face?

Try answering these questions in the following time frames.

- One-year goals
- Five-year goals
- End-of-practice goals

Making an audio-visual recording of yourself may seem intimidating. You may wonder if it is necessary. One of the reasons you are strongly encouraged to record yourself in this session is that it allows you the rare opportunity of seeing yourself. Unlike home movies, in which the emphasis may be on how you look, this recording will focus on what you say and how you say it. You will be able to see yourself as others see you and gain a different perspective on yourself. An audio-visual recording, unlike a written account, is more spontaneous, allowing you to say what is on your mind without worrying about punctuation or grammar.

○○○ *Group exercise*: The audio-visual experience
⊂⊃ *(30–90 minutes)*

Looking at oneself in pictures or on audio-visual records can be an unnerving experience that many approach with fear and others simply avoid. Having just created a record of yourself, it is a good time to discuss the experience. As a group, try to take a look at the benefits and risks of having been recorded. Each participant should independently write down all the advantages and disadvantages that the experience presents. Then going around the room, each participant should mention one plus and one minus about the exercise that has not yet been mentioned by the other participants. Keep circling the group until all the items on everyone's list have been mentioned.

Listing all the pluses and minuses on a flipchart will give participants a 'master list'. Reviewing this complete list will allow individuals, as well as the group, to make a final decision on the merits of this experience. You may find that this discussion will give you new ideas on how you can review and use your recording in the future.

Evaluation

Evaluation is the ability to make a judgement about the value of something. It entails a 'looking back'. Judgements are often made with reference to predefined criteria or standards, for example when we are assessing the value of a research report, determining whether or not a patient has achieved certain goals or monitoring and auditing the extent to which targets have been achieved within services. Evaluation is a high-level skill in both reflective practice and academic study and it is challenging because we have to face the facts. Unfortunately, the idea of evaluation can make people feel uncomfortable; it has associations with examinations, performance appraisals and assessment. The fear of being judged badly may naturally make us want to avoid it altogether.

Self-assessment or evaluation is a personal process in which we examine ourselves, frequently and over time. This is an important component of reflective practice and professional education. Whilst we can receive input from others and include their observations and opinions, ultimately we must judge ourselves. Evaluation is not meant to be self-torture for past misdemeanours. Rather, it should be future orientated; for example, it may involve finding discrepancies between what is needed and what is actually done, in order to make necessary changes. Autobiographies often contain interesting examples of self-evaluation, showing how people look back on their lives. Try reading some.

On-your-own exercise: Listening to yourself and others (*15–30 minutes*)

Play back your own or, with permission, your partner's audio-visual recording. Listen to what is said on the recording and take notes on the following.

- Beliefs/values
- Problems to overcome
- Goals for the future

 With-a-partner exercise: Learning from the past and looking to the future (*30–60 minutes*)

Review with your partner the notes that you have taken about the audio-visual recording. Ask your partner if they agree with each of the items you have put into the categories of beliefs/values, about problems to overcome, and goals for the future.

After the discussion with your partner, change any of the items if necessary. Use the rest of the time with your partner identifying the following.

- Ongoing support systems
- Ongoing strategies
- Outlook for the next year of practice

Group exercise: Closure (*30–90 minutes*)

For the last gathering of the group, it is good to look back on the experience, look forward, and look inward at the group. This session should be a time to review and acknowledge all the hard work that went into the exercises. This last session should be personalised by the group in a way that participants feel most appropriate to their experience. A celebration might be in order!

A more wide-ranging approach to developing reflective practice

As we have indicated earlier, many of the skills-based exercises in this chapter are aimed at nurses who are at the beginning of their reflective journey. However, some of you may have used earlier editions of this book, or other texts, to get started in reflection. You may now be wishing to develop your reflective practice further. For those nurses, we present some work drawn from that of Schön (1983, 1987). This outlines some attributes or characteristics of the reflective practitioner that can be used to focus your development. You may like to undertake an academic or practice-based course to help you acquire some of these characteristics, although we would suggest that they are best acquired through mentoring or coaching in practice.

Attributes of the reflective practitioner

Possessing a repertoire of experience

As a reflective practitioner, you will bring your past experience to new situations by recalling them from your repertoire of experience – recognising similarities between your previous experiences and the new one (Schön 1983). You would by this stage have a huge range and variety of repertoire and be conscious of this when bringing it to unfamiliar situations (Schön 1983). The reflective practitioner sees the new situation as something already in their repertoire to an extent – seeing similarities and differences with previous experience (Schön 1983). Throughout this, as a reflective practitioner, you will keep an open mind and each new situation contributes to the repertoire (Schön 1983).

Demonstrating artistic practice

As a reflective practitioner, you should be working towards demonstrating what is often called an 'artistic performance'. This ability enables you to see practice situations from several perspectives, not just that based on traditional knowledge sources. As an artistic practitioner, you would be using a repertoire of past experiences to consider the best way to act in a situation. According to Schön (1987), this attribute reveals the knowledge that you hold in your 'intelligent action' and thus shows your 'knowing in action' (Schön 1987).

Being able to frame problems and experiment in practice

As a reflective practitioner, you will act in a new situation as you have in others, but the new problem-solving behaviour that you now possess is a variation on the old one. You will be able to see what happened before and do what you did before. Schön expresses this as 'seeing as' you did before and 'doing as' you did before (Schön 1983). This is different from more habitual ways of practice in that you are framing and reframing problems to reshape them into an hypothesis for practice (Schön 1983). An experienced reflective practitioner follows rules that have not yet been made explicit and invents new rules 'on the spot' (Schön 1987). As s/he invents experiments to put new theories to the test, the practitioner restructures the usual theories of practice (Schön 1987) and behaves more like a researcher than an expert (Schön 1987). This is what we might see in our practice when we try out new ways of solving patient care problems that are not amenable to normal practice interventions. As you experiment to discover the consequences of your actions, the situation 'talks back' to you, allowing you to reframe the problem (Schön 1983).

Having an ability to articulate your reflective practice

As a reflective practitioner, you may be limited in your ability to put into words what you do (Schön 1987). However, in this situation you may be able to articulate the new situation 'in light of' the old one (Schön 1983). Yet, reflective practice is not dependent upon being able to articulate what is done or what it reveals about us (Schön 1987). What we are saying here is that the reflective practitioner can describe deviations in practice from the norm but not necessarily what the norm is (Schön 1987).

Having a transactional and constructivist relationship with practice

As a reflective practitioner, you will find that you begin to hold a reflective conversation with the situation at hand (Schön 1983). This is what Schön (1983) terms a transactional relationship with the unique practice situation as the professional waits for the results of experimentation to 'talk back'.

Possessing tacit knowledge

The competence of reflective practitioners is of a high-powered, esoteric nature (Schön 1983). This means that it is difficult to 'pin down' to one source or type. The reflective practitioner demonstrates connected 'anticipation and adjustment' in detecting and correcting errors in practice. This means that as you go about practice, you are constantly adjusting what you are doing. It is your tacit knowledge (Schön 1987) that enables you to act in all the above ways because it is your own individual way of knowing and is shown in the ways in which you can anticipate patient outcomes and combine your knowing in action and your smooth performance (Schön 1983).

I wonder how you feel after reading all this? It might be that you think that this is a very 'tall order', and it is. Yet, many of you, particularly those who have long experience in nursing, will be already demonstrating these attributes in your daily work. Here are some thinking points that may be of help.

Thinking activity

When next in practice, stop for a moment and consider where the knowledge for your actions comes from. Think about your experience, your 'repertoire' and how you ascertain 'clues' from practice situations that suggest a certain line of action.

We can often find several sources of knowledge for practice decisions; this supports our 'world of practice'. It is unique to us as individual practitioners, but others share the same experiences. We all 'experiment' in practice to a certain degree. One of the difficulties with this is that the practice world is full of procedures and guidelines that can limit us in the actions we take.

 Thinking activity

Consider an incident where you took action that differed from what would be considered to be the 'norm' for that situation. What prompted you to act differently? What was it in the situation that caused you to take this course of action? How did you know whether what you did was the best action (or not)?

We sometimes find it difficult to talk with colleagues about such situations – particularly if we have deviated from an established 'norm'. However, many of these 'norms' are unwritten rules or just constitute what is usually accept-able practice in a particular context. It can take quite a lot of courage to admit that you have done something differently. In fact, sometimes we are not totally aware that we have done so; it just comes 'instinctively'.

 Thinking activity

To what extent is the practice knowledge that you possess derived from practice? How much comes from more formal learning? Are there differences in the type of knowledge that comes from these two sources?

This understanding of how we gain and develop our knowledge for practice is useful in that it not only highlights the amount of understanding that we derive from our daily work, but also how very important this knowledge is. It is easy, and common, for nurses to devalue this. Reflective practice is about an awareness of where our understandings come from and a purposeful use of this knowledge. Finally, in this section, we want to say that if much of this seems to have little meaning for you at present, or if you prefer the skills-based approach outlined above, do not worry about this. We all have our own learning preferences and it may be that the 'attributes' approach will be helpful as you gain more experience and confidence in using reflection. You might also like to look at the work of Jennifer Moon (1999) who has some interesting ideas on the features of reflective practice, which suggests some attributes or characteristics of those who might fulfil this role.

Conclusion

The intention of this chapter has been to raise your awareness of the key skills and attributes that we believe underlie reflective practice and to encourage and support you as professional practitioners in facilitating and developing these skills and attributes. It is evident that skills for reflective practice are not discrete and separate elements, but are interrelated parts of a whole reflective process. While breaking down the process of reflective practice into constituent parts may be helpful as a strategy for learning and teaching, the challenge comes with combining and integrating the different elements. This is why we have introduced the wider-ranging notion of reflective practice as a set of attributes, a 'way of being' that may be more suitable for more experienced practitioners. It is important to remember that genuine reflective practice can only be developed by becoming immersed in actually doing it. This is essential for developing an approach to professional practice, or a way of thinking, whereby we constantly review our practice in order to learn and to improve standards of care. We recommend you now to Chris Bulman's final chapter where you can consider some of the practical issues involved in developing reflective skills.

Acknowledgements

This chapter draws significantly on the following unpublished work:

Atkins, S. and Murphy, K. (1993) Developing skills for profiling learning. An unpublished open learning package. Oxford Brookes University, Oxford.

Mackin, J. (1997) Reflections in the mirror of experience: understanding the ethical dilemmas of nursing practice. Unpublished doctoral dissertation and open learning package. Teachers College, Columbia University, New York.

Our sincere thanks go to Kathy Murphy and Janet Mackin for their contributions.

References

Atkins, S. and Murphy, K. (1993) Reflection: a review of the literature. *Journal of Advanced Nursing*, **18**, 1188–1192.

Bloom, B.S., Englehart, M.D., Furst, E.J., Hill, W.H. and Krathwohl. D.R. (1956) *Taxonomy of Educational Objectives, Handbook 1: Cognitive Domain.* Longman, London.

Bolton, G. (2010) *Reflective Practice: Writing and Professional Development*, 3rd edn. Paul Chapman Publishin, London.

Boud, D., Keogh, R. and Walker, D. (1985) Promoting reflection in learning: a model. In: Boud, D., Keogh, R. and Walker, D. (eds) *Reflection: Turning Experience into Learning*. Kogan Page, London.

Boyd, E.M. and Fales, A.W. (1983) Reflective learning: key to learning from experience. *Journal of Humanistic Psychology*, **23**(2), 99–117.

Brockbank, A. and McGill, I. (2007) *Facilitating Reflective Learning in Higher Education*, 2nd edn. SRHE/Open University Press, Buckingham.

Brookfield, S.D. (1987) *Developing Critical Thinkers: Challenging Adults to Explore Alternative Ways of Thinking and Acting*. Open University Press, Milton Keynes.

Brookfield, S.D. (1991) *Developing Critical Thinkers: Challenging Adults to Explore Alternative Ways of Thinking and Acting*, 2nd edn. Open University Press, Milton Keynes.

Brookfield, S.D. (1995) *Becoming a Critically Reflective Teacher*. Jossey-Bass, San Francisco.

Burnard, P. (1997) *Know Yourself!* Self-awareness Activities for Nurses. Scutari Press, Harrow.

Burrows, D.E. (1995) The nurse teacher's role in the promotion of reflective practice. *Nurse Education Today*, **15**, 346–350.

Carper, B.A. (1978) Fundamental patterns of knowing in nursing. *Advances in Nursing Science – Practice Orientated Theory*, **1**(1), 13–23.

Carper, B.A. (1992) Philosophical inquiry in nursing: an application. In: Kikuchi, J.F. and Simmons, H. (eds) *Philosophical Inquiry in Nursing*. Sage Publications, Newbury Park.

Daly, W.H. (1998) Critical thinking as an outcome of nursing education. What is it? Why is it important to nursing practice? *Journal of Advanced Nursing*, **28**(2), 323–331.

Driscoll, J. (ed) (2007) *Practising Clinical Supervision: A Reflective Approach for Healthcare Professionals*. Baillière Tindall/Elsevier, Edinburgh.

Duffy, A. (2007) A concept analysis of reflective practice: determining its value to nurses. *British Journal of Nursing*, **16**(22), 1400–1406.

Duke, S. and Appleton, J. (2000) The use of reflection in a palliative care programme: a quantitative study of the development of reflective skills over an academic year. *Journal of Advanced Nursing*, **32**(6), 1557–1568.

Durgahee, T. (1998) Facilitating reflection: from a sage on stage to a guide on the side. *Nurse Education Today*, **18**, 419–426.

Fisher, A. (1995) *Infusing Critical Thinking into the College Curriculum*. Centre for Research in Critical Thinking, University of East Anglia, Norwich.

Glaze, J.E. (2001) Reflection as a transforming process: student advanced nurse practitioners' experiences of developing reflective skills as part of an MSc programme. *Journal of Advanced Nursing*, **34**(5), 639–647.

Glaze, J.E. (2002) Stages in coming to terms with reflection: student advanced nurse practitioners' perceptions of their reflective journeys. *Journal of Advanced Nursing*, **37**(3), 265–272.

Hannigan, B. (2001) A discussion of the strengths and weaknesses of 'reflection' in nursing education and practice. *Journal of Clinical Nursing*, **10**, 278–283.

Higgs, J. and Titchen, A. (2000) Knowledge and reasoning. In: Higgs, J. and Jones, M. (eds) *Clinical Reasoning in the Health Professions*, 2nd edn. Butterworth Heinemann, Oxford.

Jarvis, P. (1992) Reflective practice and nursing. *Nurse Education Today*, **12**, 174–181.

Jasper, M.A. (1999) Nurses' perceptions of the value of written reflection. *Nurse Education Today*, **19**, 452–463.

Johns, C. (2009) *Becoming a Reflective Practitioner*, 3rd edn. Wiley Blackwell, Oxford.

Johns, C. (2011) *Guided Reflection*, 2nd edn. Wiley Blackwell, Oxford.

Johns, C. and Freshwater, D. (eds) (2005) *Transforming Nursing Through Reflective Practice*, 3rd edn. Wiley Blackwell, Oxford.

Light, G. and Cox, R. (2009) *Learning and Teaching in Higher Education: The Reflective Professional*, 2nd edn. Paul Chapman Publishing, London.

Mann, K., Gordon, J. and MacLeod, A. (2007) Reflection and reflective practice in health professions education: a systematic review. *Advances in Health Sciences Education Theory and Practice*, **14**(4), 595–621.

McGill, I. and Beaty, L. (2001) *Action Learning: A Guide for Professional, Management and Educational Development*, 2nd edn. Kogan Page, London.

Mezirow, J. (1981) A critical theory of adult learning and education. *Adult Education*, **32**(1), 3–24.

Moon, J. (1999) *Reflection in Learning and Professional Development. Theory and Practice*. Routledge Falmer, Abingdon.

Page, S. and Meerabeau, L. (2000) Achieving change through reflective practice: closing the loop. *Nurse Education Today*, **20**, 365–372.

Paget, T. (2001) Reflective practice and clinical outcomes: practitioners' views on how reflective practice has influenced their clinical practice. *Journal of Clinical Nursing*, **10**, 204–214.

Polanyi, M. (1958) *Personal Knowledge: Towards a Post-Critical Philosophy*. Routledge and Kegan Paul, London.

Ruth-Sahd, L.A. (2003) Reflective practice: a critical analysis of data-based studies and implications for nursing education. *Journal of Nursing Education*, **42**(11), 488–496.

Scanlan, J.M. and Chernomas, W.M. (1997) Developing the reflective teacher. *Journal of Advanced Nursing*, **25**, 1138–1143.

Schön, D. (1983) *The Reflective Practitioner*, 2nd edn. Jossey-Bass, San Francisco.

Schön, D. (1987) *Educating the Reflective Practitioner*. Jossey-Bass, San Francisco.

Stewart, S. and Richardson, B. (2000) Reflection and its place in the curriculum on an undergraduate course: should it be assessed? *Assessment and Evaluation in Higher Education*, **25**(4), 369–380.

Styles, M.M. and Moccia, P. (eds) (1993) *On Nursing: A Literary Celebration*. National League for Nursing, New York.

Van Horn, R. and Freed, S. (2008) Journaling and dialogue in pairs to promote reflection in clinical education. *Nursing Education Perspectives*, **29**(4), 220–225.

Wong, F., Loke, A., Wong, M., Tse, H., Kan, E. and Kember, D. (1997) An action research study into the development of nurses as reflective practitioners. *Journal of Nursing Education*, **36**(10), 476–481.

Chapter 3

Writing to learn: writing reflectively

Sylvina Tate

School of Life Sciences, University of Westminster, London, UK

Introduction

Once you have developed your reflective skills, you will realise that using this way of learning is transformative, by which I mean you will start to question and challenge accepted views of the world. Being a reflective practitioner can be viewed as thoughtful, considered and well-argued transgression. However, in order to share your new understandings you need to be able to communicate these with a wider audience: your assignment marker, your professional body, your audience, your employer, your readers, your government. To successfully do this, learning to write reflectively is the key underpinning skill.

Within this chapter, my intention is to enthuse and motivate you to engage with the process of reflective writing in a way that empowers you to take your own journey. To achieve this, I will first introduce you to the process of journalling; what it is, how to do it, the benefits of journalling and some of the blocks you may encounter. This will be supported with examples of my own work and some from students. This will be followed by exploring the nature of reflective writing by comparing it to the traditional way of academic writing. The chapter will end with an exploration of some of the professional and ethical issues you may encounter in writing reflectively.

In the spirit of authenticity, it is important to me that I share relevant aspects of myself and my own personal reflective journey to give you some understanding and insight into my choices for inclusion within this chapter. I have been teaching, facilitating and researching reflective practice for over 20 years. In every reflective group with which I have worked, there have been a range of responses to my suggestion that participants keep a personal journal. These responses range from resistance and confusion through to enthusiasm and commitment. Those of you who keep

Reflective Practice in Nursing, Fifth Edition. Edited by Chris Bulman and Sue Schutz.
© 2013 John Wiley & Sons, Ltd. Published 2013 by John Wiley & Sons, Ltd.

a journal will understand the value of recording your thoughts, feelings and experiences in the moment (or as close to the moment as is practical). However, being aware of the differing learning styles of individuals, I have no intention of limiting the nature of journalling; indeed, I hope to offer you a wide range of possibilities, freeing you as an individual to choose to engage with your own journey in a way that is personally congruent.

Having read this far through the book, I hope you have now realised that reflection is a process rather than a 'one-off' activity. I always feel slightly amused by students who commence a course and then apply to APEL reflective modules, because they have 'already done it'! I understand the motivation of reduced cost and increased time, but in many ways this indicates to me that they have learnt nothing about reflection. Being a reflective practitioner is not something you 'do', it is something you 'are'; it is your way of being – in every part of your life. Some students have reported how the process of reflection has totally transformed their lives – I take no responsibility for the positive outcome other than for introducing them to a new way of learning and facilitating their novice reflections. It is they who have engaged in the process, it is they who have identified personal areas for change, it is they who have implemented strategies to change aspects of their personal and professional life. One of the underpinning tools in this process is the maintaining of a personal journal.

I intentionally use the phrase 'personal journal' rather than 'reflective journal' for a number of reasons. Firstly, without any doubt, the journal is the personal property of the writer and no-one else. It is not written to be marked or judged. Secondly, I believe that not much reflection takes place in a journal; the journal is only the 'data collection tool'. Reflection takes place in the next phase of your journey through working with the content of your journal. I will explore this process later in this chapter.

Finally, by using the phrase 'reflective journal' I believe barriers are raised to maintaining a journal. I hear the fear in student voices as they ask questions such as: 'What does a reflective journal look like?', 'How do I do it?' and 'What is the right way?', indicating to me their need to 'get it right', to please the teacher rather than empower themselves.

As you start your journey, know that you are doing this for you; to be the best nurse that you can possibly be, while working within a range of social, financial, political and personal constraints. I share everything to support, challenge and empower you.

Your personal journal

Reflection is about 'doing' rather than 'telling', it is about first-hand knowing through 'experience' rather than second-hand knowing through reading textbooks, it is about subjectivity (you) rather than objectivity (the collective other), it is about journey (process) rather than arriving (outcome), it is about opening up to possibilities rather than a 'one size fits all' mentality. It is a heuristic[1] way of learning.

I want to be congruent to the philosophical underpinnings of reflection and as such want to open you up to possibilities rather than close you down to one way. However, as someone who has 'academic' as one of my roles, I would be reneging on my responsibilities if I did not direct you to the work of others. In doing this, please do not accept their work (including mine) as more valuable than your work; read it, consider it but please critique it and remember that it is only a recording of the author's experience which could be very different from yours for all sorts of reasons.

Where does your personal journal fit into your reflective learning?

Personal journals have been explored and described in varying ways by a range of authors (Moon 1999; Jasper 2003; Johns 2009). However, I have found that Johns (2010) is the most comprehensive and practical. It is important to understand that reflective learning cannot take place without understanding the context in which your experience has occurred, the bigger picture that is impacting on the personal. This is referred to as the hermeneutic spiral.[2] Johns (2010) suggests that there are 'six dialogical movements within the hermeneutic spiral of being and becoming' (p.27), i.e. there are six steps in the process of understanding and sharing your experiences (see Box 3.1). The first step is the keeping of a personal journal. This can be viewed as your data collection process. The other five steps refer to how you explore and understand your data.

The keeping of a personal journal is not therefore just a self-indulgent egocentric activity. If used with intention and commitment, it is the start of a challenging, insightful and transformatory process through which you will empower yourself and understand your currently unconscious behavioural and emotional patterns (we all have them). It will change how you view yourself and the world. I hope you are ready to start.

[1] Heuristic refers to experience-based techniques for learning, 'allowing pupils to learn for themselves' (*Collins English Dictionary*).

[2] Hermeneutics is the study of the theory and practice of interpretation. The hermeneutic spiral is the process of exploring your experiences by understanding its individual parts within the context of the whole, e.g. social, psychological, cultural and historical. This means you cannot understand your experiences without understanding the context of your experiences.

Chapter 3

Box 3.1   The six dialogical movements (Johns 2010)

First dialogical movement	Maintaining a journal in which you record your subjective experiences as a rich story, drawing on all your senses and accessing your inner voice to express your feelings relating to the experience
Second dialogical movement	Here you try to dialogue with your story in a more objective way. At this stage it is helpful to use a model of reflection so that you can ask the same questions of your different stories. The aim is to try and obtain personal insights from your story
Third dialogical movement	In this stage you examine your insights using external sources such as published texts, to try and gain more understanding about them
Fourth dialogical movement	The fourth movement requires you to dialogue with guides, such as your supervisor or supervision group, to check out and deepen your insights. They can help you to consider other perspectives about your story
Fifth dialogical movement	At this stage you create a narrative of your journey by pulling together your reflective insights that have occurred through the previous four movements
Sixth dialogical movement	Dialoguing with others by publication, performance or presentation with the aim of providing consensus of insights and resulting in social action

The purpose of a personal journal

I have touched on the main purpose of a personal journal which is to record your personal[3] experiences. However, I would like to focus on the purpose in a little more depth. Bolton (2010) distinguishes between the terms 'log', 'diary' and 'journal'. She suggests that a log is a recording of specific information, which is limited and predetermined. It is devoid of extraneous data. She uses the ship's log to illustrate this concept. A diary can contain anything: 'stories of happenings, hopes and fears of what might happen, memories, thought and ideas, and all the attendant feelings. It can also contain creative material: drafts of poems, stories, plays or dialogues, doodles and sketches' (p.156).

A journal, she suggests, is a diary with a purpose. This means you can include anything that pertains to the purpose of the journal. So one of the

[3] When I use the word 'personal' in the context of experiences I am referring to any experience that has happened to you, either of a personal or professional nature.

key questions that would be helpful for you to consider is: 'What is my purpose for keeping a reflective journal?'.

Exercise 1

Before you read any further, spend 10 minutes considering 'What is in it for me to keep a personal journal?'. Make a list of all the ways you believe a personal journal could benefit you.

Individuals keep journals for many reasons; some are internally motivated, such as helping to deal with a life crisis or recording details of a special time. I recall hearing a radio interview with a woman who went to live on a remote Scottish island with her husband. She became fascinated with the seals living there and to occupy her time spent a number of years keeping a journal about her observation of their behaviour. This became so comprehensive that she was eventually awarded a PhD for her work.

Other reasons may be externally motivated, for example, meeting the requirements of a course you are studying. It is increasingly common to require students to maintain reflective journals as a source of data to demonstrate having achieved learning outcomes for a module or course. I have kept three journals focused on meeting the requirements of courses: my Postgraduate Diploma in Education, my Yoga Teacher's Diploma and currently my PhD. However, external motivation may be other than a course or assessment. For example, during the Second World War a mass observation project was established with the aim of recording everyday life in Britain. Women from all walks of life volunteered to keep journals recording the 'nitty gritty' of their lives between 1937 and 1945. This information has resulted in, among other things, the publishing of several books[4] which demonstrate the richness of the data contained in personal journals.

So, regardless of whether your journal is internally or externally motivated (or both), you can make it work for you. On a personal level, I have found that my externally motivated journals have helped me in many ways beyond their intention. To give you some examples: I have identified personal beliefs, become aware of patterns of behaviour, dealt with emotions, supported myself during challenging times, considered difficult decisions, and noticed areas of stress held within my body. This experience is strongly supported in the literature.

In fact, Moon (1999) provides a very useful summary of the benefits that others have obtained from keeping a personal journal which I have summarised and added to in Table 3.1. Although I have started with Moon's

---

[4] Examples: Trustees of the Mass Observation Archives (2006) *Nella Last's War: The Second World War Diaries of 'Housewife, 49'*. Profile Books, London.

Sheridan, D. (ed) (2002) *Wartime Women: A Mass Observation Anthology of Women's Writings, 1937–1945 (Women In History)*. Phoenix Press, London.

Table 3.1   Reasons for keeping a journal (Adapted from Moon 1999)

Reason	Summary	Evidence
Process reasons		
To record experience	This is the first step in reflective learning. A practical example is the maintaining of a professional portfolio	Wolf (1980) Johns (2010)
To enhance personal ownership of learning	By dialoguing with the text and asking critical questions to develop an awareness of taken-for-granted assumptions	Jenson (1987) Johns (2009)
To engage in deep learning processes	By exploring the theory to understand your personal situation	Mortimer (1998) Jensen (1987) Berthoff (1987)
To foster reflection and creative interaction in a group	To explore possibilities through supervision group discussion	Walker (1985)
To increase self-awareness and empowerment	By increasing personal insights into personal and professional behaviour	Cooper (1991) Morrison (1996)
To enhance creativity	By helping to connect with the inner intuitive elements of the self	Christensen (1981)
Outcome reasons		
To learn from experience	Through the analysis of critical incidents, possibly using a model of reflection to interrogate the story	Flanagan (1954) Wolf (1980) Walker (1985)
To enhance other forms of learning	Supporting the research processes through reflexivity	Alvesson and Skoldberg (2009)
To understand personal learning processes	By becoming aware of your personal learning style and utilisation of that approach	Morrison (1996) Handley (personal communication, 1998)
To enhance problem-solving skills	The reflective process is a transferable skill in problem solving. You learn to analyse situations with the intention of changing your actions to achieve more positive outcomes	Jensen (1987) Grumbacher (1987) Korthagan (1988)
To develop the professional self in practice	Developing awareness of dissonance between beliefs, values and actions	Moon (1999) Johns (2009)

Table 3.1 *Cont'd.*

Reason	Summary	Evidence
For therapeutic and behaviour-changing purposes	Helping to implement changes towards personal and professional congruence	Progoff (1975) Cooper (1991)
To free up writing and the representation of learning	Often by overcoming personal blocks around writing ability	Jensen (1987) D'Arcy (1987)
To provide an alternative 'voice' for self-expression	By expressing yourself in different ways	Johns (2009) Schuck and Wood (2011)
For assessment of formal learning	A personal journal provides the data to demonstrate having met the learning outcomes	Redwine (1989)

summary, my summary subdivides the reasons into process and outcome and has added to the sources.

Starting your journal

Starting your journal will, for some of you, be the most challenging step but like any transforming process, it is a challenge that, once overcome, can lead to amazing insights and rewards. However, I am not claiming that this just happens, as if by magic. It will only produce rewards if you are prepared to invest in, and work with, the process.

So, before you write a word, you need to make a decision about the type of journal you intend to use. At the suggestion of the word 'journal', you may immediately think of writing with pen on paper and while this may be the preference of some, there are a range of options from which to choose. Possibilities that come to mind are notebooks, loose-leaf files, computers, blogs, recordings, videos. This is not meant to be a comprehensive list, rather a representation of possibilities.

Paper-based journals tend to be either in notebook or loose-leaf form. My personal choice is a bound notebook, many types of which are available. Mine are diverse in nature, varying from a blank sketchbook through to purposely designed journals with encouraging daily affirmations. Each includes personal words, extracts from books, drawings, cuttings, narratives, photographs, artefacts and pressed flowers. Their diversity of shape, size and colour sitting on my bookshelf represents my growth over the years. The truth is that when I started journalling I never gave my choice of journal a second thought, I used the first available book I found. Some of you may prefer to use a consistent type of book, and thus the result in 5 years' time will be much more aesthetically pleasing (if this is important to you).

Entries from journals can be used as evidence to support subsequent learning, but I acknowledge the difficulty in finding entries at a later date. The plus side is that the re-reading always brings surprise and pleasure. Personally, I love the feel of touching and holding something concrete in my hands and scribing spontaneously with a pencil.

It has been suggested to me that when using a paper journal, I only write on the left-hand page, leaving the right hand for future reflective thoughts, insights, cross-referencing to appropriate theory and analytical conclusions. I have found this a very helpful discipline in connecting theory to insights and stories.

Bolton (2010, p.160) uses:

'... a loose-leaf folder that can hold all sorts of shapes and sizes – A4 sheets of written (handwritten and typed), letters, newspaper cuttings, journal papers, pictures, and all sorts of other items. And I like to write with a 2b pencil with a rubber on the end: I think I like the idea of being able to rub out my writing, though I never do; I also like the whisper a soft pencil makes on the page.'

Alternatively, technology may be your preferred way of keeping a journal. Johns (2010, p.29) writes:

'Before we can reflect, we must first access our experiences. I sit at the computer wondering how to write my stories. Remembering a moment ... the look on her face, a word said, a tear, the feeling I feel inside, a sad smile, a smell of curry, a picture on the wall, the dance of the trees outside the window ... so many signs to trigger my story.'

Johns is a prolific author on reflective practice and his journalling directly onto the computer must make it easier to edit and incorporate relevant aspects into his books. This may be a useful strategy if, as a student, you are keeping a journal with the purpose of writing an assignment for a course or module. You may find it quicker to retrieve specific entries as evidence for your learning and it will save time if you use the 'cut and paste' facility on your computer.

I am aware of some courses that require students to maintain a reflective blog. This generally happens between defined groups of students and allows dialogue to occur between interested parties. My question relating to this is about the type of entry a person will record when they are aware it is for public consumption. It may inhibit you for a number of psychological and ethical reasons. Recording our deeply personal thoughts and feelings for public consumption may leave us feeling very vulnerable if the qualities of trust and unconditional acceptance are not established within the group. Revealing this type of information can only feel safe when the fear of judgement is absent.

Even if you feel safe within your group, there is always the fear that other non-group individuals may be able to hack into the server and access your contributions. A greater fear, linked to this, is the potential for contributions to 'go viral' and end up on the wider internet.

From a long-term perspective, there is always the potential for your contributions to be used as evidence in any future disciplinary and professional misconduct hearings relating to yourself and others. Even when deleted from the computer, entries can be retrieved by relevant experts.

Finally, I have a friend who believes (quite erroneously) that he cannot write, so he records his journal on his mobile phone, taking photographs to combine with his narrative as he walks to work. It works for him.

In essence, the type of journal you keep is very personal, connected to your preferences and choices. It needs to be your choice.

Exercise 2

Spend 10 minutes considering the following questions.

- How are you feeling about keeping a reflective journal?
- Are any internal messages emerging to discourage you?
- What have been your past experiences relating to writing?

Make a note of your responses in your journal (I hope you have one now!).

Blocks to writing

Having chosen your type of personal journal, you now need to start writing in it. This can be a huge block for some people.

Rolfe *et al.* (2001) suggest that our previous experiences of writing have probably been to provide evidence to others of what we have learnt, rather than as a process to help us learn about ourselves. They quote Allen *et al.* (1989) who define two concepts of 'learning to write' and 'writing to learn'. When keeping a personal journal you are 'writing to learn' and they suggest that the assumptions listed in Box 3.2 are associated with 'writing to learn'.

In reading Box 3.2, you will notice that the emphasis is all about learning. It is not about spelling, grammar, syntax, paragraph construction or essay construction. Your personal journal is for your eyes only and will never be judged, marked or commented upon. It is the first step in your reflective learning process. It is the opportunity to play with thoughts, feelings and explore your experiences. In fact, depending upon your preferred way of learning, it may be more meaningful and less intimidating to make journal entries that don't utilise words and grammar. An example of such a technique that I have used is mind mapping (Buzan 2002): no grammar, no sentences and lots of pictures!

However, if you find you still feel a block to starting a journal, Julia Cameron (1992), in her book *The Artist's Way*, suggests tools that can

> **Box 3.2   Assumptions associated with writing to learn (Rolfe _et al._ 2001)**
>
> Writing is a process through which content is **learned** or **understood**
>
> Writing skills are primarily **thinking** skills
>
> Writing is a process of **developing an understanding** or coming to know something
>
> Writing is a **dialectical, recursive process** rather than linear or sequential
>
> **Higher order conceptual skills** can only evolve through a writing process in which the writer engages in an active, ongoing dialogue with themselves and others. **Learning and discovery** are purposes as important for writing as communication
>
> Different disciplines utilise different conceptual processes and thus have **different standards for writing**. Students can best learn writing within their own discipline while writing for a specific purpose such as an assignment
>
> **(My emphasis is in bold text.)**

help to overcome this. She explains that our left, logical, categorical brain is our greatest critic. Based on stored messages from the past, it is constantly telling us how we can't write coherently, that our grammar is poor and our spelling weak, etc. This is the source of most writing blocks. In contrast, the right brain, which she calls the 'artist brain' (p.13), is our inventor. It is creative and holistic, thinks in patterns and can be utilised to overcome our blocks.

She believes that the best way to overcome writer's block is to engage in what she calls 'morning pages'. Put simply, these are three pages 'of long-hand writing, strictly stream-of-consciousness', written as soon as you wake every morning. There is no wrong way of doing them, they are not meant to sound coherent or intelligent, just whatever comes into your mind. She suggests that you do this for 12 weeks and initially do not read them or share them with anyone. You may find that when you do read them, they may sound 'negative, frequently fragmented, often self-pitying, repetitive, stilted or babyish, angry or bland – even silly sounding' (p.10). 'Good!' Julia exclaims. 'All that angry, whiny, petty stuff that you write down in the morning stands between you and your creativity. Worrying about the job, the laundry, the funny knock in the car, the weird look in your lover's eye – this stuff eddies through our subconscious and muddies our days' (p.11). The message is to just get it on the page and out of your subconscious.

So if you are one of those people who believe they can't write, I challenge you to take up Julia's suggestion and contract with yourself to write three pages every day for 3 months. You may be amazed at the outcome.

Content

I hope that by now you are ready to take up the challenge to start your journey and engage with your personal journal. The next question you need to address is: 'What do I include in my journal?'. As Bolton (2010) indicated, a journal is a diary with a purpose so before you start your journal, you really need to be very clear about its purpose. Three common purposes are:

- to provide evidence to meet assessment criteria
- to research self
- for personal development.

I will now explore each of these in more detail.

To provide evidence to meet assessment criteria

If you are undertaking a course and are required to keep a journal and write a reflective account as part of your assessment, then you need to look at the learning outcomes for the course or module. In doing this, ask yourself 'What am I required to demonstrate as part of this assessment?'. To illustrate the process, I will use an example from a module of study that I deliver as part of an undergraduate degree (Box 3.3).

Box 3.3   Linking personal journals to module learning outcomes

---

The assignment: a reflective study

The reflective study is designed to enable you to demonstrate what you have achieved during the year in relation to learning outcomes 1 and 2, using a reflective framework.

Learning outcomes 1 and 2

On successful completion of the module you should be able to:

1. critique aspects of the unconscious within the therapeutic relationship
2. evaluate reflectively the role of your unconscious within the therapeutic relationship as experienced in clinic and class.

Consider and make a note of the type of entries you might include in your journal if you were undertaking this assignment.

Of course, there are no right or wrong answers in relation to the above question, but the reflective study does need to include personal information demonstrating how insights have developed about your own unconscious processes and how this has impacted on your therapeutic relationship with clients.

Your personal journal may include any or all of the following information.

- Incidents when interacting with clients.
- Incidents when interacting with peers in class.
- Times when you have felt attracted to or repelled by others.
- Times when you have felt inadequate.
- Times when you have felt really good.

The focus of your entries would be the therapeutic relationship, detailing your behavioural patterns that may potentially indicate an as yet unconscious message, which you want to explore, understand, challenge and change through the use of reflection.

The assignment detailed in Box 3.3 is submitted at the end of the module. During the period that the module runs, each student is part of a group of peers who, with a facilitator, function as a peer supervision group. The students are required to keep a journal focusing on the puzzling, challenging and enchanting experiences of their therapeutic relationships from both the module and their supervised practice (Johns' first dialogical movement).

Following their personal reflections on their journal entries, they choose an incident, pattern or issue about which they would like to develop a deeper understanding (Johns' second dialogical movement). Each student then presents their experience to their peer supervision group and receives reflective feedback from both peers and facilitator (Box 3.4) (Johns' fourth dialogical movement). This feedback is then reflected upon and incorporated into a narrative, the purpose of which is to demonstrate achievement of the learning outcomes (see Box 3.3).

I recognise that each assignment is specific to each module, with differing time scales, focus and learning outcomes. However, the process illustrated in the above example will be useful to follow for any reflective assignment.

In summary:

- identify the learning outcomes for the module
- journal regularly, focusing on the subject relevant to the learning outcomes
- review your journal monthly to notice patterns, anxieties or positive practice
- meet regularly with a peer supervision group to present and explore issues that concern you. (I suggest that you read Chapter 6 on clinical

Box 3.4   Example of presentation feedback

Areas for reflection

Thank you for presenting your case which was very relevant to you and your self-esteem issues. Your area for exploration was 'I always feel that whatever I do is not good enough'.

You were honest and open in answering the questions of your peers and were able to recognise some of your patterns, e.g. that you always see yourself as lacking compared to your older sister, always wanting to prove yourself.

I suggest that you reflect on some of these questions.

- In relation to your client, you stated 'I felt I had let her down'. Is this a common thought for you? Why do you feel responsible? Why could you not challenge your supervisor? Why could you not explain honestly to your client what your intention was, i.e. that you had limitations within your skills but rather than refer her immediately (and give her no treatment), you were going to give her a treatment that may or may not work but was worth trying and that if it did not work then you would refer her?
- You said you feel you are a 'Jack of all trades'. Could you reflect on why you don't stick with one 'trade'? Is this because you **believe** that you will never be an expert or is it because you have not found your passion, or is it something else?
- You said you wanted feedback from your client. Can I ask you to reflect on your questioning skills, e.g. instead of asking 'How was it for you?' (a general and global question), you ask more specific questions, e.g. 'Is your neck feeling more comfortable?'
- When receiving feedback, can you see that for what it is – feedback on a technique that will help you to grow and develop, rather than a personal attack? It is interesting that I have just watched the film 'The Voyage of the Dawn Treader'. In it, Lucy (the younger sister) wants to be like Susan (the older sister). It would be worth going to see it to find out the advice that Aslan gives to Lucy – very profound.
- Could you keep an appreciation diary? Writing in it at the end of the day all the positive things that happened. It is interesting that I did it as a one-off last night, looking back over my life, and I was able, without even thinking too much about it, to produce two pages of things I am grateful for. I am sure you could do the same.
- Can you read the theory around 'Countertransference and projection' and read up about 'Drivers', especially 'Try harder ' and 'Please others', and consider what changes you can implement to diminish these.

Chapter 3

supervision before engaging in this process. It is essential that ground rules are agreed and adhered to.)
- provide each other with constructive and supportive feedback
- use the feedback and personal reflection to enhance your assignment.

To research self

Reflection can be used as a research tool for dissertations at all academic levels. A number of my undergraduate students have chosen this approach. Their motivation is to understand, develop or modify aspects of their therapeutic relationships. Their focus has included qualities such as loving-kindness and empathy, and skills such as the use of Heron's (2001) six-category interventions, listening skills and self-disclosure.

Researching self requires a similar approach to writing a reflective study or essay, whereby you are both researcher and researched. The main differences are the time scale and the depth of your reflections. An immediate response may be that you query the validity of and the bias within such an approach. If this is the case, a useful book to consult would be *Reflexive Methodology* (Alvesson and Sköldberg 2009). Alvesson and Sköldberg claim that 'interpretation-free, theory-neutral facts do not, in principle, exist' (p.1). They also suggest that critics of empiricism 'claim that culture, language, selective perception, subjective forms of cognition, social conventions, politics, ideology, power and narration all, in a complicated way, permeate scientific activity' (p.2).

Reflective research has two basic characteristics: reflection and careful interpretation. These qualities require a constant dynamic between the external and internal, drawing on externally located theory to explore explanations and reflecting on internal processes to consider 'the perceptual, cognitive, theoretical, linguistic, (inter)textual, political and cultural circumstances that form the backdrop to – as well as impregnate – the interpretations' (Alvesson and Sköldberg 2009, p.9), previously referred to as the hermeneutic spiral. I will try to demonstrate this process by using an example from a student (to whom I will give the pseudonym of Jane).

Jane was a final-year undergraduate student. She had previously worked in an occupation which was not patient focused and wished to research and develop her use of empathetic skills while dealing with her patients.

Jane's first step was to research the concept of empathy. What did the literature suggest were the qualities of empathy? From the literature, using the work of Rogers (1961), Egan (2002) and Burnard (1997), she developed a log to quickly record information related to her use of empathetic skills while dealing with each individual patient. The log was completed immediately after finishing her intervention with each patient (Box 3.5).

Box 3.5 Model (log) for developing patient-centred empathy

Date:	Identifier:	Sex:	Culture:	Age:
Was I empathetic and able to understand how the patient felt? Rogers: • Was I warm and genuine? • Open and non-defensive? • Did I 'prize' the patient, i.e. unconditional positive regard?				
Egan: • Did I practise the technique of mirroring back what the patient said, e.g. 'You feel … (emotion) because of … (experience or behaviour)? • What were the patient's emotions? • Did I respond accurately to the patient's feelings, emotions and moods? • Did I respond accurately to key experiences and behaviours in the patient's stories?				
Burnard's listening zones • Zone 1: 'outer' total focus on patient • Zone 2: inner thoughts on reality • Words, timing, volume, pitch, intensity, • Non-verbal communication • 'Disturbances' that blocked listening?				
Key words used by patient. • What were the core messages?				
Did I: • Ask 'why' questions? • Interrupt and stop listening? • Make assumptions? • Use the words 'could, should, need'? • Make judgements? • Give advice? • What did I learn about me? • What was uncomfortable?				
Clinical intervention • Was it comfortable for the patient? • Did I observe safety, body language and ask for feedback from the patient as I performed the intervention?				

At the end of each day, the logs were expanded upon within her journal. At a later date, Jane finally constructed a reflective analysis of each situation, using five distinct areas which she used to focus her analysis of each situation. She named these areas: Preparation, Living, Uncovering, and Reflection and Future.

- *Preparation*: related to the time prior to meeting her patient.
- *Living*: related to her actual experiences of interacting with her patient.
- *Uncovering*: occurred when she re-read her journal entries and was able to stand back from the event and ask herself reflective questions about it.
- *Reflection*: was her response to the questions she asked of herself.
- *Future*: this was when she identified ways in which she could act differently.

These headings enabled Jane to focus on all aspects of her patient interaction and explore relevant questions to help her reflect upon her experiences with the intention of identifying her personal patterns. Once she identified her patterns, she considered alternative ways of acting to modify her behaviour within future interventions. By using this technique, she was able to filter out her other interventions and focus on thoughts, behaviours and feelings relevant to empathetic behaviour.

When her data collection period was completed, Jane was able to analyse her interventions both quantitatively and qualitatively. Table 3.2 provides a summary of her empathetic interventions over the period of her research.

By using this chart, Jane was able to see how her skills had developed over time with each patient. What she was not able to do was to develop awareness and understanding of her internal processes. This required her to dialogue with her story (Johns' second dialogical movement), explore her experiences through the literature and with her critical friends (Johns' third dialogical movement) and her research supervisor (Johns' fourth dialogical movement), before developing her deep personal insights which were identified within her dissertation (Johns' fifth dialogical movement).

This process resulted in an in-depth reflection for each patient encounter. Each reflection was summarised to access personal insights and future action. An example of Jane's personal reflection relating to one patient encounter is provided in Box 3.6.

Within her dissertation, in response to the reflective analysis (Box 3.6), Jane wrote:

'Once I became conscious of my behaviour around negative emotions I began to observe my feelings, especially when I felt

Table 3.2   End of research summation of information obtained from completed logs (see Box 3.5)

Patient no.	Sex	Culture	Rogers: warm, genuine	Burnard: zones, active listening	Egan model	Intervening with intention
			Affective	Cognitive	Behavioural	Behavioural
1. 1st visit	F	Indian	Yes	No	No	N/A
2. 1st visit	F	S. Africa	Yes	No	No	Yes
3. 1st visit	F	Saudi	Yes	No	No	N/A
3. 2nd visit	F	Saudi	Yes	No	No	Yes
3. 3rd visit	F	Saudi	Yes	Yes	No	Yes
3. 4th visit	F	Saudi	Yes	Yes	Yes	N/A
4. 1st visit	F	Brazilian	Yes	Yes	No	Yes
4. 2nd visit	F	Brazilian	Yes	No	No	Yes
4. 3rd visit	F	Brazilian	Yes	Yes	Yes	Yes
5. 1st visit	F	Turkish	Yes	No	No	N/A
5. 2nd visit	F	Turkish	Yes	Yes	No	No
5. 3rd visit	F	Turkish	Yes	Yes	Yes	Yes
6. 1st visit	M	English	Yes	Yes	Yes	Yes

threatened. I noticed that when I had disagreements I blocked hearing and listening. I began to change this pattern by detaching from my own emotions, stopping my judgements and assumptions in order to hear and actively listen to what they were saying. Instead of reacting defensively, I attempted to stay with their emotions, asking direct and open questions to gain an understanding of what they were feeling.'

Reflection on self and its associated identification of personal development points can be both a very challenging and rewarding process. Without the support of a trusted supervisor, one may feel a sense of lack or inadequacy. However, on completion of her dissertation, Jane felt unburdened and developed a great sense of personal understanding and acceptance. As a result of this, she was able to present her work at a reflective practice conference, thus completing the sixth dialogical movement described by Johns (2010).

Box 3.6   A reflective analysis on a patient encounter

Patient 4 A difficult day

Brazilian lady, 46, presenting with tennis elbow and hot flushes.

Preparing

She had the last appointment of the day and I was feeling very tired especially as I had handed in my business plan at lunch time. Before meeting the patient, the supervisor warned me that she had been beaten up by her husband over the Christmas period and had a burst ear drum and lots of bruising.

Living

I did not feel in a good space and felt the tension building inside me so I pushed the patient's problems away from me. I sensed that we both put up boundaries. She did not want to go over the events and just wanted treatment as normal. I was relieved. I only had enough energy to finish my day in clinic. I felt overwhelmed hearing about her problems and was conscious that I could not connect with her, which I was disappointed about but resigned myself that this was a difficult day. Both our moods reflected each other. I made a mental note to practise qigong* every day to help me focus better on my patients.

Uncovering

- Why did I not want to listen to the patient, especially as she needed a lot of support?
- Did I feel uncomfortable because I did not want to ask prying questions?
- Was I too tired to listen to her at the end of the day?
- Did lack of experience in the patient-centred approach hold me back from being open to her?
- What about boundaries? Was I protecting myself because she was emotionally vulnerable and hurting deep inside?

Reflecting

She was a vulnerable person and more so because she was starting the menopause. By placing her in 'context' both socially and psychologically,

Contd.

I could understand her situation. I made a note of these injuries in her file although the incident had been reported to the police and she had been checked out at the hospital.

Due to lack of consultation skills, I held back empathy as I felt there were too many emotions behind this clinical encounter. I didn't have the energy to listen especially to negative emotions. I put up my defences to cover my lack of experience. Also I recognised that I do not know how to deal with negative emotions because they were not tolerated in my large family. We were always expected to be positive.

Future: To focus on staying open and being non-judgemental. Give the patient space and time to talk, go into their frame of internal reference, learn to recognise when I am putting up blocks to listening.

*Qigong is a system of exercises originating from China. It is claimed that with regular practice, you can increase awareness and focus. It was Jane's method of supporting herself.

For personal development

Keeping a journal for your own personal growth and development gives you the freedom to be as creative as you wish. According to Bolton (2011, p.18), 'expressive and explorative writing is really a process of deep listening, attending to some of the many aspects of the self habitually blanketed during waking lives'. This type of writing is primarily about process rather than product; it is about your own personal journey. However, that journey can have very positive outcomes. Bolton claims that the process can produce significant therapeutic effects including self-understanding and well-being, alleviation of stress and anxiety, dramatically supporting positive self-image and increasing communication skills.

Because of the nature of this type of journal, I have no access to any other person's content. However, even if I did, as a statement of authenticity and a demonstration of commitment, I would still use my own experiences as an example. This is not meant to represent 'the way of doing it' but rather to provide you with something that I hope will inspire you to start your own personal journal as a way of committing to becoming the person you wish to be.

My journal contains details of remembered dreams, feelings, actions, personal development workshops I have attended, things and situations that have inspired or troubled me, and the activities I have engaged in as well as everyday mundane events. Not only do I include words in my journal but also drawings, mind maps, photographs, artefacts, poems (my own generally) and inspiring quotes from books I am reading. In fact, I include whatever my heart connects with – I do not limit myself.

The first example consists of two drawings I made during a meditation workshop 5 years ago, the first at the beginning of the day and the second at the end of the workshop (Box 3.7). They were drawn from the heart rather than the mind; by this, I mean I connected with my feelings and allowed those feelings to be depicted as a drawing of a tree, while suspending censure and self-judgement.

However, words can be equally powerful. I vividly remember every moment of my day whenever I reread this entry.

This entry can be explored from a number of angles. The idea of spirituality, what is it? What does it mean for me? The role of acceptance and 'flowing'? The idea of 'being' instead of 'doing' and how this impacts on me. My connection with nature and the idea of noticing a 'lime tree speaking to me'?

Box 3.7   Drawings from my journal

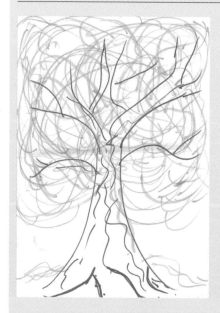 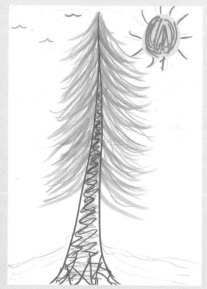

Tree 1 – a representation of myself at the beginning of the day. Well grounded, free flowing, expansive, vibrant and energetic.

Tree 2 – a representation of myself at the end of the day. Focused, strong, growing to the light – connected, boundaried, contained and directioned

These two drawings are a constant reminder of how a day of meditation impacts upon me.

Chapter 3

Exercise 3: Drawing yourself as a tree

Before you start this activity, make sure you will not be disturbed for about 30 minutes. Take your journal and some crayons, felt tips or pencils (choose whichever you prefer) with you.

- Find a place that nurtures you; it can be inside or outside in nature.
- Make yourself comfortable in a sitting position, with your eyes closed or open (whichever is most comfortable for you).
- Take a slow deep breath in through the nose. Imagine this breath is going into and expanding your heart.
- Gently breathe out, imagining that your breath is leaving your heart through the front of your chest.
- Continue this process for about 5 minutes.
- Notice how you are feeling.
- After approximately 5 minutes, gently open your eyes (if they were closed) but still try to keep your connection with your heart.
- Taking your crayons, draw a tree in your journal that represents how you are feeling at this moment. Place no judgements on your tree. It can be any colour, any shape, any size … it is your tree.
- When you have finished your tree, observe it, trying not to make critical judgements, and make a note in your journal of what you notice about the qualities of your tree.

This exercise can be repeated whenever you feel the urge.

Journal entry 26th June 2010

'It started when I woke up feeling tired and in pain with my neck. Had a coffee and went back to sleep. Woke at 8.50–10 minutes after the conference coach had left!! I decided there was nothing I could do about it so decided to shower and have a leisurely breakfast. The day was hot and I decided to walk to the conference. I was walking through the woods and felt peaceful and connected – I remembered that my name means 'wood nymph' – I listen to, touch and connect with the trees. As I walk up the lime grove – a tree 'speaks' to me – very loudly – I connect with it and it gives me messages … messages … messages … I photograph it from all angles to capture the messages … my heart opens more … I feel connected … whole and truly at peace with myself and the world.'

It helped me to understand my need for activities to enhance my connection to my inner self and resulted in me commencing a meditation teacher's course and a PhD (based on reflection, of course).

Messages from the trees

Related to the above entry, I took many digital photographs of the lime trees over the period of about an hour. I chose to print them out and place them in my journal, leaving space between each one to write about the picture and explore the message.

I then reconnected with a different photograph on a daily basis, looking at it, wondering about it, noticing aspects of the tree, reflecting on my observations and trying to understand and explore what learning I could take from the tree.

Below are two examples of my photographs and my reflective thoughts relating to them. You will notice that these reflections lead to other questions rather than solutions. This is normal. Reflection is an ongoing continual process. If you end up with more questions than answers, you are probably on the right track.

Renewal and healing

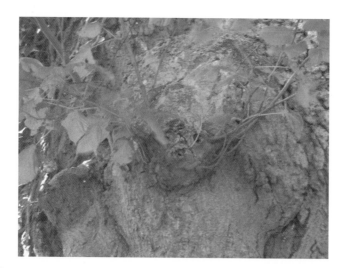

I write:

'At some point in the past this tree has lost a branch. I notice how the bark has grown to protect the wound. The tree has healed and renewed itself. I also notice that from this wound new growth has emerged. It confirms for me how pain, wounds and damage can lead to new understandings, new insights, and new growth. In fact, most of my psychological growth has happened through pain and wounds. I wonder why it is that this occurs for so many but for others it destroys them?'

Different things to different people: perspective and role

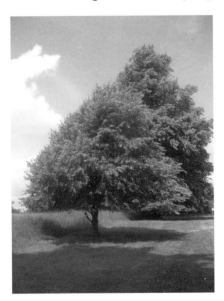 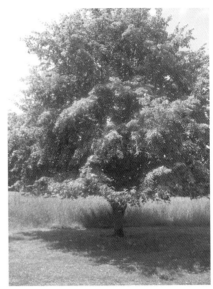

I write:

'this is the same tree – how different! It reminds me that different people have different perspectives on the same thing. It also reminds me that I present different personas in different roles – no-one knows the whole me – does being authentic mean changing this? Should I be 'what I am is what you get'? I sometimes think that this is an excuse for not considering others and giving them respect. The tree is different from different perspectives and it is OK!'

My photographs and journal entries are providing me with questions about issues that I need to work with in a reflective way. I am still (over a year later) exploring what the quality of 'authenticity' means for me. Reflective writing rarely gives quick or absolute answers.

Poetry

Poetry is not something I have in the past connected with. I would never call myself a poet or even have ambitions to be one. However, to my utter surprise, I have in my journal a collection of poems which have 'emerged from me' without any planning, thought or intention. Often this happens after a period of meditation. Below is one such poem which I have titled 'April Rebirth'. I see it as a representation of my struggle with darkness and my desire to realise my potential. My meditation had been focused on being open to new directions. I finished my meditation and wrote this poem without thought or intention. I believe it came from a part of me that is not my rational mind.

April Rebirth

April sun spotlights my piece of heaven on earth.
Plants painting the earth yellow, green, white, violet and pink.
Green algae revealed on ornaments and paving flags.

Buddha looks grubby and faded.
I wonder how he would feel if he was real?
Unconcerned I would imagine.
I spray him with gray shiny paint – he looks good.

Nataraj dances on his demons, dull and neglected.
Reminding me to control my ego.
Washed and polished, arbour swept and plants pruned.
Look at magnificent me, he shouts …

Totem pole lies sadly in the soil – dirty, faded and dejected.
Cleaned, washed, painted and renewed.
Vibrant message of story pervades the garden … My story.

Greenhouse cold, dirty and full of discarded hanging baskets
*   and pots.*
Few survived the winter and my neglect.
Each returned to the earth through composting – completing their
*   life cycle.*
Glass cleaned, floor swept, disinfected – ready to support another
*   cycle.*

Seeds; teeny, tiny, dried, inconsequential spots, full of potential.
Planted, watered, warmed and fed.
Teeny, tiny green shoots burst from darkness to light.
The start of their journey towards realising their potential.

Me … sweeping, cleaning, painting, pruning, planting, potting,
*   watering, nurturing,*
Tidying and putting into order.
Continue my journey towards realising my potential.

The April sun spotlights my aches and pains; physical and
*   emotional.*
With light comes shadow; with joy comes pain.

I am ordering, connecting, noticing and feeling.
I wish it was so easy to sort out me, to reach my destination of
*   realised potential.*

On a different level, I wrote the following haiku following a facilitated 'story telling' workshop. The outcome was the production of a personal 'fairy tale' the essence of which was distilled into 17 syllables following the haiku pattern of 5:7:5.

Listen to your soul
Speaking only from your heart
Listen feel and flow

Personal journeys can be creative, inspiring and lead to very deep learning. Of course, your journal will be very different from mine simply because it is yours. That is what will make it unique and very special.

What is reflective writing?

I have so far focused on the journalling process, the process of collecting your data by recording your experiences with particular emphasis on your thoughts, feelings and behaviours, the first dialogical movement described by Johns (2010). However, many of you will be reading this book as a resource prior to undertaking reflective work. I will therefore now focus on Johns' fifth dialogical movement, whereby you create a narrative of your journey by pulling together the reflective insights that have occurred as a result of working through the previous four movements. This will result in the production of a reflective narrative which will meet the requirements of your goal, be it a module assignment, an article for publication, evidence for your portfolio or just for personal pleasure.

Before constructing your narrative, you need to know the criteria against which it will be measured or assessed. These criteria can be externally or internally generated. If you are undertaking an assignment, you will have been given criteria against which it will be marked. An article for publication will have associated journal criteria offered as author's guidelines; portfolio entries will have guidelines from the relevant professional body. Even if you are producing the narrative as a personal exercise, you need to have identified your goals before you start. Box 3.8 gives examples of assessment criteria. These are associated with the assignment described in Box 3.3.

One of the biggest mistakes students make when writing a reflective assignment is their style of writing. This type of error tends to fall into one of the following two common mistakes: using a traditional, objective, rational, third-person approach or using a stream-of-consciousness approach. Neither approach is 'wrong' given the correct context.

Box 3.8   Examples of assessment criteria

- Demonstration, through cyclical critical reflection, of the relationship between your growing understanding and perception of yourself and your role as a practitioner.
- Demonstration of developing understanding and application of the models and theories presented in the curriculum.
- Evidence of self-appraisal and re-evaluation of how you might now understand your different behaviours, and how you might facilitate clients and/or colleagues differently. This needs to include exploration of your own underlying assumptions, attitudes and values.
- Structure and coherence of the essay.
- Presentation and referencing according to course guidelines.

Exercise 4

Take some time to identify the assessment criteria for your narrative. Once you identify the criteria, read them carefully.

Ask yourself the question 'Do I understand what is being asked of me?'.

If there are aspects that you do not clearly understand, identify ways of developing clarity.

List five ways that could help you develop clarity.

Choose one of the five possibilities and implement an action plan.

However, the first approach is more appropriate for non-reflective, traditional academic essays and the second more suited to journal entries or novel writing. Writing reflectively lies between these two approaches.

Probably the best clarification of what exactly constitutes reflective writing has been produced by Jennifer Moon (2004), who has written about this and developed some very helpful online resources. I would strongly recommend that you access this resource prior to commencing your first piece of reflective writing. Her comparison between writing styles is reproduced in Table 3.3.

I recognise that we all learn in differing ways so if you are the type of person who learns through practical exercises or visual representation, I would strongly recommend that you visit the following website: www.cemp.ac.uk/people/jennymoon/reflectivelearning.php, where you will find examples of reflective writing. By reading examples of what a reflective narrative is or is not, you will be able to understand what to avoid and what to aim for.

Table 3.3   A comparison of report or essay writing and reflective writing

Undergraduate report/essay writing	Reflective writing
The subject matter is likely to be clearly defined	The subject matter may be diffuse and ill structured
The subject matter is not likely to be personal	The subject matter may be personal
The subject matter is likely to be given	The subject matter may be determined by the writer
The purpose of this kind of writing is set in advance, usually fairly precisely in a title/topic	There may be purpose, but it is more in the nature of a 'container' or direction, not a precise title that predicts the outcome
Most of the ideas drawn into an essay/report will be predictable and will be determined by the subject matter	Ideas will be drawn into reflective writing from anywhere that the writer believes to be relevant. What is drawn in will be determined by the sense being forged by the writer
There will be a conclusion	There may be a conclusion in that something has been learnt, or there may be recognition of further areas for reflection
Essays/reports are more likely to be 'one off' – finished and handed in	Reflective writing may be part of a process that takes place over a period of time
There is likely to be a clear structure of introduction, discussion and conclusion	There is not necessarily a clear structure other than some description at the beginning and some identification of progress made. Structures, such as questions to prompt reflective activity, may be given
The writing style is likely to be relatively objective – probably without use of the first person	The writing style is likely to be relatively subjective, with involvement of the first person
An essay or report is usually intended to be a representation of learning	The intention underlying reflective writing is likely to be for the purpose of learning
An essay/report is likely to be the product of a thinking process, tidily ordered	Reflective writing usually involves the process of thinking and learning, and it is therefore not necessarily 'tidy' in its ordering

Moon (2004) identifies four stages in the development of reflective writing. To help you understand the differences, I have partly (relating to stages 1 and 4) reproduced one of her exercises below.

Exercise 5: **The park – an exercise in reflective writing (Adapted from Moon 2004)**

Below are two accounts of an incident in a park. They are recounted by 'Annie' who was involved in the incident herself. They are written as different versions of the same event to demonstrate different levels of reflective writing.

The intention of this exercise is to help you identify the differences between descriptive and reflective writing.

1. First read account 1 and ask yourself the following questions, making notes in your journal.
   - Does this account cover the issues for reflection and note their context?
   - Is there evidence of standing back from the event to mull over the situation?
   - Is there any recognition that, over time, the frame of reference with which an event is viewed can change?
   - Is there any critical awareness of one's own processes of mental functioning?
   - Is the incident noted from multiple perspectives?
   - Is there any evidence of self-questioning?
   - Are the views and motives of others taken into account?
   - Is there any recognition of the role of emotion in shaping the account?
   - Is there any recognition of the influence of prior experience and thoughts on current behaviour?
   - Have any points for learning been noted?
2. Next, read account 4 and ask yourself the same questions, noting these answers in your journal.
3. Once you have completed these two stages, I suggest that you meet with a group of peers who have also completed the exercise to discuss your findings.
4. You can then compare your findings with the comments made by Jennifer Moon, which you can find in Appendix 1 to this chapter.

The park (1)

I went through the park the other day. The sun shone sometimes but large clouds floated across the sky in a breeze. It reminded me of a time that I was walking on St David's Head in Wales – when there was a hard

Contd.

and bright light and anything I looked at was bright. It was really quite hot – so much nicer than the day before, which was rainy. I went over to the children's playing field. I had not been there for a while and wanted to see the improvements. There were several children there and one, in particular, I noticed, was in too many clothes for the heat. The children were running about and this child became red in the face and began to slow down and then he sat. He must have been about 10. Some of the others called him up again and he got to his feet. He stumbled into the game for a few moments, tripping once or twice. It seemed to me that he had just not got the energy to lift his feet. Eventually he stumbled down and did not get up but he was still moving and he shuffled into a half sitting and half lying position watching the other children and I think he was calling out to them. I don't know.

Anyway, I had to get on to get to the shop to buy some meat for the chilli that my children had asked for their party. The twins had invited many friends round for an end-of-term celebration of the beginning of the summer holidays. They might think that they have cause to celebrate but it makes a lot more work for me when they are home. I find that their holiday time makes a lot more work.

It was the next day when the paper came through the door – in it there was a report of a child who had been taken seriously ill in the park the previous day. He was fighting for his life in hospital and they said that the seriousness of the situation was due to the delay before he was brought to hospital. The report commented on the fact that he had been lying unattended for half an hour before someone saw him. By then the other children had gone. It said that that several passers-by might have seen him looking ill and even on the ground and the report went on to ask why passers-by do not take action when they see that something is wrong. The article was headed 'Why do they "Walk on by"?'. I have been terribly upset since then. James says I should not worry – it is just a headline.

The park (4)

It happened in Ingle Park and this event is very much still on my mind. It feels significant. There was a child playing with others. He looked hot and unfit and kept sitting down but the other children kept on getting him back up and making him play with them. I was on my way to the shop and only watched the children for a while before I walked on. Next day it was reported in the paper that the child had been taken to hospital seriously ill – very seriously ill. The report said that there were several passers-by in the park who had seen the child looking ill and who had done nothing. It was a scathing report about those who do not take action in such situations.

Contd.

It was the report initially that made me think more deeply. It kept coming back in my mind and over the next few days I began to think of the situation in lots of different ways. Initially I considered my urge to get to the shop – regardless of the state of the boy. That was an easy way of excusing myself – to say that I had to get to the shop. Then I began to go through all of the agonising as to whether I could have misread the situation and really thought that the boy was simply overdressed or perhaps play-acting or trying to gain sympathy from me or the others. Could I have believed that the situation was all right? All of that thinking, I now notice, would also have let me off the hook – made it not my fault that I did not take action at the time.

I talked with Tom about my reflections on the event – on the incident, on my thinking about it at the time and then immediately after. He observed that my sense of myself as a 'good person who always lends a helping hand when others need help' was put in some jeopardy by it all. At the time and immediately after, it might have been easier to avoid shaking my view of myself than to admit that I had avoided facing up to the situation and admitting that I had not acted as 'a good person'. With this hindsight, I notice that I can probably find it easier to admit that I am not always 'a good person' and that I made a mistake in retrospect than immediately after the event. I suspect that this may apply to other situations.

As I think about the situation now, I recall some more of the thoughts – or were they feelings mixed up with thoughts? I remember a sense at the time that this boy looked quite scruffy and reminded me of a child who used to play with Charlie. We did not feel happy during the brief period of their friendship because this boy was known as a bully and we were uneasy either that Charlie would end up being bullied, or that Charlie would learn to bully. Funnily enough, we were talking about this boy – I now remember – at the dinner table the night before. The conversation had reminded me of all of the agonising about the children's friends at the time. The fleeting thought/feeling was possibly something like this: if this boy is like one I did not feel comfortable with – then maybe he deserves to get left in this way. Maybe he was a brother of the original child. I remember social psychology research along the lines of attributing blame to victims to justify their plight. Then it might not have been anything to do with Charlie's friend.

So I can see how I looked at that event and perhaps interpreted it in a manner that was consistent with my emotional frame of mind at the time. Seeing the same events without that dinner-time conversation might have led me to see the whole thing in an entirely different manner and I might have acted differently. The significance of this whole event is chilling when I realise that my lack of action nearly resulted in his death – and it might have been because of an attitude that was formed years ago in relation to a different situation.

Contd.

This has all made me think about how we view things. The way I saw this event at the time was quite different to the way I see it now – even this few days later. Writing an account at the time would have been different to the account – or several accounts that I would write now. I cannot know what 'story' is 'true'. The bullying story may be one that I have constructed retrospectively – fabricated. Interestingly, I can believe that story completely.

From this exercise you will have identified some of the key characteristics of reflective writing. However, to incorporate these into your writing and to help with the development of your assignment, it may be helpful to ask yourself key questions. However, the downside of this is the time it will take you to identify a useful list of questions. However, do not despair! Fortunately for us, various authors have constructed and published their own lists of key questions which they call 'reflective models'. One or more of these models may be of use to you.

Models of reflection

A commonly used phrase comes to my mind when recommending models of reflection. That phrase is 'the map is not the territory'. By this, I mean that it is important to recognise the difference between a representation of something and the real something. So, for example, if I show you a model car you would have no difficulty recognising it as a representation of a car rather than an actual car. So it is with reflective models. They are a representation of the reflective process, a map to guide you, as novice reflectors, through the reflective process. They are based on the experiences and research of the specific authors who developed these models from differing perspectives and for different purposes. Each is slightly different but each follows the common principles of the reflective process.

Because each of us is an individual with different preferred ways of thinking and learning, I would strongly recommend that you familiarise yourself with a range of models, then select the model with which you connect and use this as a structure for your questioning. None is intrinsically better than another, although each has its advantages and disadvantages. Examples of some of the more popular models can be found in Appendix 2 (Gibbs 1988 Adapted by Tate) and Chapter 9 (Gibbs 1988 Adapted and Updated by Bulman; Driscoll 2007; Johns 2010). However, a word of caution; as Johns (2009) indicates, models:

'... may offer the novice reflective practitioner a way to access the breadth and depth of reflection, yet it is folly to think that they can "know" reflection in this way. These models threaten to impose an understanding of reflection that skims the surface of its potential depth and subtlety. At some point the practitioner must break free from the shackles of models in order to swim within the vast ocean of life' (p.6).

Are you ready to jump into the shallow end of the swimming pool? Before you do, a few words of warning!

Professional responsibilities

As someone who is either studying to become or is already a qualified healthcare professional, I would like to demonstrate the explicit link between reflection and your professional accountability.

Your professional code for standards of conduct, performance and ethics (Nursing and Midwifery Council 2008) identifies four overall professional responsibilities.

1. Make the care of people your first concern, treating them as individuals and respecting their dignity.
2. Work with others to protect and promote the health and well-being of those in your care, their families and carers, and the wider community.
3. Provide a high standard of practice and care at all times.
4. Be open and honest, act with integrity and uphold the reputation of your profession.

I believe that these are standards that every nurse and midwife can wholeheartedly agree with. However, for all sorts of reasons, you may find that at times your actions are not always congruent with your beliefs. This is not something unique to nurses. Argyris and Schön (1974) identified these differences as 'theories in action' (what you actually do) and 'theories of action' (what you believe you do). Often they are different.

Schön (1983, p.42) explored these concepts further in his seminal book on becoming a reflective practitioner, using the concepts of 'the high hard ground' and the 'swampy lowlands'. If you imagine yourself on a mountain looking down on a swamp, you can see 'the big picture' and it is very easy to map your way through the swamp. This he equates to the position of researchers and policy makers. However, if you find yourself in 'the swamp', the way forward can be difficult and challenging. He equates the 'swampy lowlands' with our everyday professional practice, going on to describe it as: 'where situations are confusing "messes" incapable of technical solution'. He concludes by suggesting that 'the problems of the high ground, however great their technical interest, are often relatively unimportant to clients or to the larger society, while in the swamp are the problems of greatest human concern'. I connect with this imagery of working in a healthcare situation and trying to meet the sometimes conflicting needs of patients, relatives, colleagues, other professionals and my employers while maintaining my professional standards.

The pressure of these conflicting demands can ultimately lead to stress-related illnesses, compassion fatigue and eventually burnout, aspects of which I have personally experienced. Keeping a reflective journal is one thing you can do to support yourself. Ideally, the support of a clinical supervisor and a peer supervision group will help you to understand your patterns, identify ways of acting differently and support you in implementing changes. Through my own reflections and subsequent supervision, I eventually came to understand the role of my unconscious 'Please others' and 'Be perfect' drivers in my responses to pressure, i.e. being unable to say 'no', trying to 'rescue' everyone, becoming single-minded and seeing things only from my viewpoint (Stewart and Joines 1987).

To take just one of these responses, 'rescuing everyone', if you are familiar with the theory of transaction analysis, you will recognise the consequences of that behaviour. Those being rescued don't learn from their mistakes and therefore cannot grow and develop. They become dependent on their rescuer but also blame their rescuer when things do not turn out as anticipated. They do not learn to take responsibility for their decisions and actions. This does not represent an equal, respectful and collaborative working relationship. This outcome was dissonant with my personal values and beliefs and the realisation resulted in me implementing changes in my behaviour. However, please remember that deep patterning takes a long time to alter, so be kind to yourself when you find yourself falling back into familiar ways of responding (as I did). Just keep journalling, reflecting and implementing changes – eventually the pattern shifts. It is a life-long journey of learning and changing initiated by you, which is why I suggested at the beginning of this chapter that being reflective is not something you 'do'; rather it is something you 'are'.

Underpinning your journalling there always needs to be a question, and as a nurse or a nursing student, your questions need to be related to becoming and being the best nurse possible. Some examples could be as follows.

- What kind of nurse do I wish to be?
- How do I make the care of people my first concern, treating them as individuals and respecting their dignity?
- How do I provide a high standard of practice and care at all times?
- Do I work with others to protect and promote the health and well-being of those in my care, their families and carers, and the wider community?
- Do I act in a way that is congruent with my beliefs and values?
- What are my professional strengths and limitations?

In engaging in this process, you will be supporting and valuing yourself, identifying professional development needs, providing evidence for your professional development portfolio and improving your professional practice.

One of the key concepts in any caring situation is the therapeutic relationship. According to the Registered Nurses Association of Ontario (2006), there are seven prerequisite knowledge bases required for an effective therapeutic relationship: background knowledge; knowledge of interpersonal and developmental theory; knowledge of diversity influences and determinants; knowledge of person; knowledge of health/illness; knowledge of the broad influences on health care and healthcare policy; and knowledge of systems. These are underpinned by four personal capacities: self-awareness, self-knowledge, empathy, awareness of boundaries and limits of the professional role (p.20). Each of these knowledge bases and capacities can be developed and refined through the use of reflective practice. You can learn about these concepts from a theoretical perspective by reading about them. However, the only way you can embody them and learn about them from your experiences is to reflect upon them, hopefully through personal reflective supervision groups.

As a professional practitioner, you are required to follow the code of conduct of your professional body, putting your client and their needs at the centre of your practice in a sensitive and humanistic way. The question for you is: can you afford to not engage in reflective practice as a means of learning, abiding by best practice and being supported in a very demanding role?

Ethical considerations

At the beginning of this chapter I stated quite categorically that your personal journal is for your eyes only. However, as a member of a professional body, you are required to abide by its code of conduct. As such, there are ethical considerations of which you need to be aware when writing in your journal. Probably the most obvious and relevant ethical issue is your requirement for patient and colleague confidentiality. Specifically:

- you must respect people's right to confidentiality
- you must ensure people are informed about how and why information is shared by those who will be providing their care
- you must disclose information if you believe someone may be at risk of harm, in line with the law of the country in which you are practising (Nursing and Midwifery Council 2008).

To abide by this, you should never refer to any other individual involved in your experiences by their actual names. Nor should they be recognisable from your descriptions. A commonly used technique in maintaining confidentiality is the use of pseudonyms.

Another issue to be aware of is related to professional misconduct. If you decide to share your journal entries with others, either informally or formally during a supervision session, please remember that the person you share with also has a responsibility to practise within their professional code of conduct. This means that consequences may ensue if your code of conduct has been contravened in any way.

Finally, and especially if you keep your journal on a computer, remember that the Data Protection Act (1998) applies to you. The Nursing and Midwifery Council has a data protection policy which can be found at www.nmc-uk.org/Privacy-and-terms-of-use/Data-protection/Data-protection-policy/.

Exercise 6:   **Ethical considerations**

Consider the following questions.

- What aspects of your code of conduct do you need to consider when starting your journal?
- With whom are you likely to share your journal entries?
- How will you maintain confidentiality and anonymity within your journal?
- Do you need to know more about the Data Protection Act 1998, and if you do, what are you going to do about it?

Conclusion

This chapter has introduced you to the idea of reflective writing as a method of deep, self-directed learning. In becoming a reflective practitioner, you will be empowered by developing increasing self-awareness, learning from your mistakes, and challenging and changing your practice in relation to your professional responsibilities, ethical considerations and moral obligations.

I hope I have challenged your perceptions about journalling and motivated you to 'give it a go'. As Jasper (2008) stated in the conclusion to this chapter in the previous edition:

> For many nurses I have worked with, the act of journalling brought reflective practice alive and made it, if not an everyday conscious activity, then certainly a regular one. Many have found that journalling enabled them to see the task of constructing a professional portfolio as a dynamic activity rather than an onerous, retrospective, dust-gathering chore'.

I would concur with her conclusion and add that it can be empowering, transformative and life changing too.

Are you ready to take the first step on your journey?

Chapter 3

References

Allen, D.G., Bowers, B. and Diekelmann, N. (1989) Writing to learn: a reconceptu-alisation of thinking and writing in the nursing curriculum. *Journal of Nurse Education*, **28**(1), 6–11.

Alvesson, M. and Sköldberg, K. (2009) *Reflexive Methodology: New Vistas for Qualitative Research*, 2nd edn. Sage Publications, London.

Argyris, C. and Schön, D. (1974) *Theory into Practice: Increasing Professional Effectiveness*. Jossey-Bass, San Francisco.

Berthoff, A. (1987) *Dialectic Notebooks and the Audit of Meaning*. Boynton/Cook Publishers, New Hampshire.

Bolton, G. (2010) *Reflective Practice: Writing and Professional Development*. Paul Chapman Publishing, London.

Bolton, G. (2011) *Write Yourself: Creative Writing and Personal Development*. Jessica Kingsley Publishers, London.

Burnard, P. (1997) *Effective Communication Skills for Health Professionals*, 2nd edn. Stanley Thornes, Cheltenham.

Buzan, T. (2002) *How to Mind Map*. Thorsons, London.

Cameron, J. (1992) *The Artist's Way: A Spiritual Path to Higher Creativity*. Tarcher/Putnam, New York.

Christensen, R. (1981) "Dear Diary": a learning tool for adults. *Lifelong Learning: The Adult Years*, **5**(2), 4–5, 23.

Cooper, J. (1991) Telling our own stories. In: *Stories Lives Tell: Narrative and Dialogue in Education*. Teachers College Press, New York.

D'Arcy, P. (1987) Writing to learn. In: Fulwiler, T. (ed) *The Journal Book*. Heinemann, New Hampshire.

Data Protection Act (1998) www.legislation.gov.uk/ukpga/1998/29/contents

Driscoll, J. (2007) *Practising Clinical Supervision*, 2nd edn. Baillière Tindall, London.

Egan, G. (2002) *The Skilled Helper. A Problem-Management and Opportunity-Development Approach to Helping*, 7th edn. Brooks/Cole, California.

Flanagan, J.C. (1954) The critical incident technique. *Psychological Bulletin*, **51**(4).

Gibbs, G. (1988) *Learning by Doing: A Guide to Teaching and Learning Methods*. Further Education Unit, Oxford Polytechnic, Oxford.

Grumbacher, J. (1987) How writing helps physics students become better prob-lem solvers. In: Fulwiler, T. (ed) *The Journal Book*. Heinemann, New Hampshire.

Heron, J. (2001) *Helping the Client*, 5th edn. Sage, London.

Jasper, M. (2003) *Beginning Reflective Practice*. Nelson Thornes, Cheltenham.

Jasper, M. (2008) Using reflective journals and diaries to enhance practice and learning. In: Bulman, C. and Schutz, S. (eds) *Reflective Practice in Nursing*, 4th edn. Blackwell Publishing, Oxford.

Jensen, V. (1987) Writing in college physics. In: Fulwiler, T. (ed) *The Journal Book*. Heinemann, New Hampshire.

Johns, C. (2009) *Becoming a Reflective Practitioner*, 3rd edn. Wiley-Blackwell, Oxford.

Johns, C. (2010) *Guided Reflection*, 2nd edn. Wiley-Blackwell, Oxford.

Korthagen, F. (1988) The influence of learning orientations on the development of reflective teaching In: Calderhead, J. (ed) *Teachers Professional Learning*. Falmer Press, London.

Moon, J.A. (1999) *Reflection in Learning and Professional Development*. Kogan Page, London.

Moon, J.A. (2004) *A Handbook of Reflective and Experiential Learning*. Routledge Falmer, London.

Morrison, K. (1996) Developing reflective practice in higher degree students through a learning journal. *Studies in Higher Education*, **21**(3), 317–332.

Mortimer, J. (1998) *Motivating Student Learning Through Facilitating Independence: Self and Peer Assessment of Reflective Practice – An Action Research Project*. SEDA, London.

Nursing and Midwifery Council (2008) *Standards of Conduct, Performance and Ethics for Nurses and Midwives*. Nursing and Midwifery Council, London.

Progoff, I. (1975) *At a Journal Workshop*. Dialogue House Library, New York.

Redwine, M. (1989) The autobiography as a motivational factor for students. In: Warner Weil, S. and McGill, I. (eds) *Making Sense of Experiential Learning*. SRHE/Open University Press, Buckingham.

Registered Nurses Association of Ontario (2006) *Establishing Therapeutic Relationships*. Registered Nurses Association of Ontario, Ontario, Canada.

Rogers, C. (1961) *On Becoming a Person*. Houghton Mifflin, New York.

Rolfe, G., Freshwater, D. and Jasper, M. (2001) *Critical Reflection for Nursing and the Helping Professions*. Palgrave, Basingstoke.

Schön, D. (1983) *The Reflective Practitioner*. Basic Books, New York.

Schuck, C. and Wood, J. (2011) *Inspiring Creative Supervision*. Jessica Kingsley Publishers, London.

Stewart, I. and Joines, V. (1987). *TA today*. Lifespace Publishing, Nottingham.

Walker, D. (1985) Writing and reflection. In: Boud, D., Keogh, R. and Walker, D. (eds) *Reflection: Turning Experience into Learning*. Kogan Page, London.

Wolf. J. (1980) Experiential learning in professional education: concepts and tools. *New Directions for Experiential Learning*, **8**, 17.

Useful websites

Moon, J.A. Resources for use with reflection or learning journals.
www.cemp.ac.uk/people/jennymoon/reflectivelearning.php
Moon, J.A. Defining and improving the quality of reflective learning.
www.cemp.ac.uk/people/jennymoon.php/

Appendix 1   The park: comments on the quality of reflection (Adapted from Moon 2004)

The park (1)

- This piece tells the story. Sometimes it mentions past experiences, sometimes anticipates the future but all in the context of the account of the story.
- There might be references to emotional state, but the role of the emotions on action is not explored.

- Ideas of others are mentioned but not elaborated or used to investigate the meaning of the events.
- The account is written only from one point of view – that of Annie.
- Generally ideas are presented in a sequence and are only linked by the story. They are not all relevant or focused.
- In fact, you could hardly deem this to be reflective at all. It is very descriptive. It could be a reasonably written account of an event that could serve as a basis on which reflection might start, though it hardly signals any material for reflection – other than the last few words.

The park (4)

- The account is succinct and to the point. There is some deep reflection here that is self-critical and questions the basis of the beliefs and values on which the behaviour was based.
- There is evidence of standing back from the event, of Annie treating herself as an object acting within the context.
- There is also an internal dialogue – a conversation with herself in which she proposes and further reflects on alternative explanations.
- She shows evidence of looking at the views of others (Tom) and of considering the alternative point of view, and learning from it.
- She recognises the significance of the effect of passage of time on her reflection, e.g. that her personal frame of reference at the time may have influenced her actions and that a different frame of reference might have led to different results.
- She notices that the proximity of other, possibly unrelated events (the dinner-time conversation) has an effect either on her actual behaviour and her subsequent reflection – or possibly on her reflective processes only. She notices that she can be said to be reconstructing the event in retrospect – creating a story around it that may not be 'true'.
- She recognises that there may be no conclusion to this situation – but that there are still things to be learnt from it.
- She has also been able to reflect on her own process of reflecting (acted metacognitively), recognising that her process influenced the outcome.

Appendix 2   Gibbs' reflective cycle (Gibbs 1998, adapted by Tate)

Description of the experience (what happened?)

Record your description at or close to the time of the experience (use your journal and date entries).

- Describe what happened (sometimes called the critical incident) in your own words using the first person.
- Try to write as objectively as possibly as if you were observing the event.
- How did you act during the experience?
- What were your thoughts during the experience?
- Try not to make judgements at this time. Record any insights as part of the experience.

Recording your feelings (what were you feeling?)

Record the feelings you were aware of during the experience, in detail at or close to the time, to begin to recognise your patterns.

- How did you feel, i.e. emotions (positive and negative) and other thoughts?
- At what point in the experience did the emotion start?
- Did you notice any physical symptoms associated with the emotion?

At a later time, return to your descriptions and recorded feelings and in your journal complete the next four sections. You may link experiences together if you begin to see patterns.

Evaluating the experience

Evaluation is about measurement against some sort of implicit or explicit standard to conclude what went well and what did not. It is important to try and evaluate components of the experience rather than the whole experience.

- Why did I interpret the situation in the way I did?
- What other interpretations might there be?
- Why did I act/intervene the way I did?
- What were the consequences of my actions for myself/others involved?
- How are negative feelings/assumptions holding me back?
- How did positive feelings influence what happened?
- How did negative feelings and fears influence what happened?
- What assumptions did I make, about myself, about others?
- What did others involved do, think, feel?

Analysis of the experience

Analysis of the component parts and exploring them from different angles to find out how you could have responded differently.

- What might I have done differently? What might have been the outcome?
- How might I put aside the features that are holding me back?

- What do I need to learn more about, and how will I learn it? (This includes background reading)
- How can I apply new learning and strategies?

Conclusion about the experience

Having identified a range of options, you now have more information on which to make a judgement. Without detailed analysis and honest exploration, it is likely that learning opportunities will be lost.

- What have I learned from the experience (about self, others, issues)?
- How has my understanding developed?
- How will I apply it another time?
- What do I need to work on – and how will I work on it?

Action plan

This is where you produce a plan to act differently.

- What is your goal?
- What steps do you need to take to achieve your goal?
- What resources do you need to achieve your goal?
- What is the time frame for each of these steps?
- What will be the outcome of each step?

Chapter 4
Reflecting in groups

Bernadette Carter
Department of Nursing, University of Central Lancashire, Preston, UK

Introduction

> 'Never doubt that a small group of thoughtful, committed citizens can change the world.' (Margaret Mead, 1901–1978)

Margaret Mead's insistence that people should not underestimate their capacity to instigate change and create better futures feels like an apposite mantra to guide reflective practice. It is a sentiment to which nurses should instantly feel aligned. It is a good place to start this chapter as it brings to the fore the power inherent in effective group reflection.

Reflective groups have a huge potential to help nurses critically consider their everyday practice regardless of the practice setting, specialty, role, level of experience or expertise. Working together in a reflective group opens up new opportunities for learning that are simply not available to nurses reflecting on their practice in a more solitary manner. Whilst group reflection can bring substantial benefits to the group members and to their care and work, it is by no means a simple solution.

Reflective group work is now used extensively within nursing (across different settings, specialties and for a range of different purposes) and one of its primary functions is to develop the capability and/or competence of the participants as there is a growing demand for an increase in productivity and efficiency, risk reduction and other benefits to the organisation. One benefit which is largely overlooked is the potential enhancement of well-being that can result from engagement in effective, reflective groups.

Although initially viewed with a degree of scepticism and as a cost-cutting exercise (Rolfe et al. 2001), reflective groups are different from, but no less resource intensive than, other approaches to reflection

Reflective Practice in Nursing, Fifth Edition. Edited by Chris Bulman and Sue Schutz.
© 2013 John Wiley & Sons, Ltd. Published 2013 by John Wiley & Sons, Ltd.

and supervision. Although groups incur a cost through the need for skilled facilitators (who in turn require skilled supervision), White and Winstanley (2006) suggest that they are more cost efficient than one-to-one supervision.

Groups have potential. They have the potential to challenge practice, bring about change, support the acquisition of new skills and knowledge, challenge practice, be emancipatory, empowering and transforming. However, groups have equal potential to go wrong. Whilst effective groups may result in energising and enthusing members, ineffective groups may simply fizzle away. Perhaps, more worryingly, ineffective groups may, amongst other things, pool ignorance, damage morale and result in a 'there's no point to trying' attitude.

Most of the reflective groups that are presented in the nursing and health literature fall into three broad categories: groups whose fundamental purpose is the enhancement of students' knowledge, skills and professional identity; groups where the focus is on clinical supervision and professional advancement of qualified practitioners; and groups that are convened for the purpose of practice development. Of course, these three categories are not exclusive and inevitably there is overlap, and some reflective groups would not fit easily within any of them. Arguably, one category which does not appear in the literature is what I would term the 'guerrilla group', a group which spontaneously and informally arises, reflects on a specific issue and then disbands.

In this chapter, reflective group work is explored in terms of some of the wider changes that are occurring in the context of professional learning. The challenges and benefits of reflective group work are examined in relation to the creativity, imagination and anxiety they can engender and in terms of the use and abuse of power. Some of the issues and artistry associated with facilitating a successful reflective group are addressed. Particular points are illustrated with experiences drawn from both being a member of, and being a facilitator of, reflective groups.

Work-based learning, organisational learning and learning organisations

Gherardi (2003) provides an inspiring way of thinking about knowledge acquisition within the workplace when she proposes that 'knowledge as an end in itself motivates people and organizations' (Gherardi 2003, p.352). By moving away from seeing knowledge purely as something instrumental that has to be acquired to remain competitive or competent, she suggests that it has its own worth and value. Gherardi's concept of 'knowing as desiring' is a refreshing way of approaching practice-based learning as it suggests we can tap into this existing willingness to learn. In recent years, the potential for harnessing the 'situated learning' that occurs in 'communities of practice' (Lathlean and Le May 2002, p.624) has been highlighted and this has also been recognised by Wenger (2000), Sheehan (2011) and Berry (2011). As Mann *et al.* (2009, p.227) note: 'Situated learning in communities of practice embraces the notion of culture and the creation of professional practice that crosses disciplinary barriers'. There has been a commensurate shift to capitalise, and make more explicit, the learning that occurs in groups.

Abma (2007, p.199) emphasises the way in which situated learning is context bound in relationships between people, and that this 'implies an intimate connection between knowledge and action'. Group work and peer support can reinforce this contextual connection for practitioners throughout the different stages of their professional growth and learning. As Walsh *et al.* (2002, p.236) note, reflection can enable 'clinicians to see anew the environment in which they work and envisage how it could be different'. Although Walsh *et al.* are talking specifically of clinicians, the same holds true of nurses working in management, education and research.

The acceptance that there is a connection between the setting and the context in which learning takes place underpins, to a greater or lesser degree, the recent interest in both work-based learning (WBL) and the notion of learning organisations. Williams (2010) emphasises how the current economic climate and the pressures on all resources mean that 'work-based learning is likely to come under increased scrutiny as a potential solution'. However, despite the benefits associated with WBL, it is 'only useful if it is both vital and rigorous' (Burton 2004, p.200). Flanagan *et al.* (2000) warn that ensuring that work-based learning is effective is challenging. The assumption that learning is synonymous with change, as Gherardi (2001, p.131) points out, 'ignores the fact that many organisational changes occur without any learning taking place, and – vice versa – that learning processes may not give rise to change'. Dewar and Walker (1999) note that there can be dissonance between the educational philosophy of work-based learning and how it is actually delivered. Effective work-based learning is predicated on supportive organisational structures, for example through nurse managers who help 'develop a learning culture in their workplace' and who 'ensure that skilled facilitation is provided to support staff with critical reflection and effecting changes in practice' (Williams, 2010).

Whilst work-based learning and situated learning can occur as isolated pockets of activity within an organisation, the notion of learning organisations extends the activity of learning throughout the organisation. O'Connor and Kotze (2008, p.174) propose that within learning organisations the emphasis is on 'proactive organisational development, a stretch towards the future and a strategic process' with the result being 'generative learning and increased capacity to take effective action'. Group reflection is one learning activity that has the potential to contribute significantly to development of a learning organisation.

Chapter 4

Groups to support reflection, learning and supervision

Groups range from very informal groups to ones which are more structured and purposive and from hierarchical ones to more democratic, equitable and co-operative groups. Reflective group working as a means of developing an individual's abilities, skills and knowledge mirrors other shifts in thinking. A common reason for reflective groups to form is to provide a forum for supervision. Traditionally, supervision and supervisory practices have been viewed from a somewhat essentialist perspective such as that proposed by Maggs and Biley (2000, p.192), who propose that supervision can 'develop competence in practice, protect the patient/client and provide structured support for the professional'. However, more recently, authors have questioned such a process-oriented, hierarchical approach to supervision (Shanley and Stevenson 2006), which 'implies a linear progress towards the practically perfect practitioner' (Stevenson 2005, p.520). Stevenson suggests that supervision meetings should be replaced by 'egalitarian consultation meetings' (ECMs) in which a dialogic approach is adopted allowing practitioners to share radical ideas about practice development. This more egalitarian approach has huge resonance for all types of reflective groups as it genuinely respects the grounded knowledge that the practitioner brings to the discussion.

Developing professional expertise and knowledge through group reflection can occur in many ways, for example, within the practice setting (embedded as part of practice), within an academic setting (embedded within modules and other learning opportunities) or blended across practice and academic settings. Heiskanen (2007, p.370) notes that increasingly 'expert knowledge is seen as shared, distributed and contextualised' and this can be supported through the use of reflective group work in nursing.

Online reflective groups

Whilst most reflective groups meet face to face, there is also potential in exploiting the benefits of newer technologies such as web conferencing, synchronous and asynchronous e-reflection groups (see, for example, Rocco 2010). There is huge potential capacity for online groups to extend communities of practice across institutional, geographical, cultural, political and social borders. Cassidy (2011), for example, demonstrates how online communities can promote knowledge construction and enhance collaboration for nurses practising mental health care in remote rural areas.

However, although e-groups offer considerable advantages in terms of extending communities of practice, they still rely on people relating to each other. Social relations are every bit as important in online groups as in face-to-face groups and, as Lee-Baldwin (2005) notes, 'social dynamics within groups play an important role in facilitating cognitively in depth levels of reflective thinking'. Experience shows that encouraging these relational links to be made – for example, through initial introductions and ongoing inquiries about the members as individuals rather than disembodied contributors of text – is crucial to effective e-groups. Knowing who you are reflecting with is essential if reflections are to be truly meaningful.

Reflecting face to face

Face-to-face reflective group work can be undertaken in a variety of different ways, for example, through action learning sets, reflective 'start and finish' project groups, clinical supervision groups and 'guerrilla groups'. Although these different formats could also work online, most of the evidence reflects examples from face-to-face meetings.

Action learning sets (ALS), a style of group working (Mumford 1996), have gained in popularity in nursing, and Douglas and Machin (2004) discuss their value in interdisciplinary collaborative working. Action learning sets can provide the reflective setting in which learners seek solutions though a 'cycle of identifying and implementing courses of action, monitoring the results, refining the action, testing again …' (Stark 2006, p.24). Action learning sets and similar reflective groups have been adopted within nursing in education and practice settings for developing clinical leadership skills (Hardacre and Keep 2003), management skills (Booth et al. 2003), the strategic skills of nurse consultants (Young et al. 2010), developing nursing practice (Garbett et al. 2007; Hardy et al. 2007; Rivas and Murray 2010), implementing the Modern Matron (Dealey et al. 2007), and end-of-life care (Hewison et al. 2011). In each of these studies, the group-based reflective element has been crucial to the personal and professional development of individuals and their practice.

Clinical supervision within reflective group-based or team-based sessions is firmly embedded as a practice and there is now a more extensive literature which explores the benefits and disadvantages of it as an approach. Lindgren et al. (2005), for example, discuss its use within pre-registration training, whereas other authors have explored its value for hospice nurses (Jones 2003, 2006) and its use within intensive care settings (Lindahl and Norberg 2002), renal and urological nursing (Kilcullen 2007), psychiatric settings (Saarikoski et al. 2006; Buus et al. 2011) and the acute hospital (O'Connell et al. 2011).

Situated learning and reflective group thinking often spontaneously arise within the workplace, leading to what I have termed 'guerilla group reflection'. In a guerilla group, a reflective opportunity is seized because it is almost impossible to resist. For example, a group which is convened for a different and not necessarily reflective purpose may be confronted by a situation which stimulates an episode of intense reflective activity, which has an effect on the people within the group who leave the guerilla group with more insight. Critics might contest the notion of a guerilla

Chapter 4

group, arguing that their informal constitution does not properly achieve reflective group status. However, these are some of the most interesting groups to be part of, as these very tightly framed periods of reflective activity can be powerful, valuable and effective. Members of guerilla groups seize reflective moments and turn these to their advantage. Recently, whilst working in a group of three people during a mandatory training session, our conversation intensified and became more reflective and our personal investment in the dialogue increased. Although not perfectly aligned to the activity we were supposed to be focused on, our reflective topic was relevant, intriguing, stimulating and almost irresistible. We pursued it. As we focused down on issues, shared experiences, sought to understand our own positions and assumptions, and those held by other people, we gained insights. This reflective group arose, was active and disbanded itself, within about 25 minutes. For me, this transitory group created a powerful episode of reflective activity and I have continued to reflect upon, respond to and take actions based on the dialogue that occurred in the group.

Group working: challenges and benefits

'The challenge in nursing education is to create fruitful conditions for a learning encounter between the student's own life world and knowledge in theory and practice.' (Ekebergh 2011)

Creating fruitful conditions

Whilst Ekebergh (2011) is talking specifically about students, her words have resonance for all nurses. Group working has the potential to create Ekebergh's fruitful conditions. However, despite the advantages inherent in group reflection, it is necessary to have insight into the challenges and difficulties that can result from this more engaging, dialogic and potentially democratic approach to reflection. Some of these challenges are summarised in Box 4.1.

Reflective group work opens up opportunities for group members to learn in different ways, for example, through developing empathy about patients' experiences through the sharing of stories or developing a stronger sense of moral purpose through the way in which another member of the group positions themselves. Individuals within a group can offer different experiences and ideas (Bold 2008; Holmlund et al. 2010) and, as Winship and Hardy (1999, p.312) note, 'many heads are better than one'. Peer support, peer feedback and a democratic sharing of experience can be nurtured within a group (Rolfe et al. 2001), and deeper learning and enhanced reflective capacity can occur (Bold 2008).

Another important aspect of reflective groups is that they can challenge the learning styles of students. In her study, Hanson (2011, p.298)

Box 4.1   Overview of the benefits, risks and challenges of group work

Benefits

- Group reflection can encourage a democratic sharing of ideas.
- Group reflection can encourage more ideas to develop and flourish.
- Using imagination and creativity in reflective groups can open up new ways of thinking and suggest new solutions.
- Group reflection can offer benefits to nurses at all stages of their careers.
- Group reflection can promote a sense of professional identity.
- Group reflection promotes peer support which can provide mutual facilitation.
- Groups where membership is heterogeneous can generate greater insights into organisational culture and practice.
- Group supervision may be perceived as less threatening for individuals than one-to-one reflection sessions.
- Groups where participants are team members can result in greater cohesion within the team's work setting.
- Group reflection may more effectively promote a sense of shared professional identity and professional competence than can be achieved in one-to-one reflective sessions.
- Group work creates increased opportunities for participants to listen attentively and learn from other group members

Risks

- Group work takes reflection into a more public domain than one-to-one reflection and this can mean that some participants may feel exposed and vulnerable.
- Group work requires everyone to 'act well'; where this does not occur, care needs to be taken to ensure that this is effectively managed.
- In groups utilising creative approaches, participants who perceive themselves to be less creative than other members can feel overwhelmed.
- Passive or active misuse or abuse of power is detrimental to group dynamics.
- Group reflection may cause anticipatory anxiety.
- Group work can be uncomfortable at times.
- Group work may result in participants experiencing vicarious distress.

Contd.

Chapter 4

Challenges

- The facilitator needs to be skilled in managing group dynamics.
- The facilitator has to be skilled and attentive to ensure that all group members feel safe.
- The facilitator needs to ensure that the aims of the group have been negotiated by all members of the group and that these are clear, explicit and shared.
- The facilitator should ideally be working towards making themselves redundant within 'their' group.
- The facilitator's role is skilled and can be challenging and facilitators benefit from support and debriefing.
- A supportive group environment requires active effort from the participants and facilitator.
- Group time needs to be protected and groups should start and end on time
- Confidentiality and anonymity need to be considered especially when practice is discussed.

focused on undergraduate students undertaking early childhood studies and noted that 'it takes time to make the transition from passive recipient of knowledge to active participant within the learning process'. Reflecting within a group definitely requires an active engagement in, and contribution to, learning.

The use of imagination within reflective practice groups can help create and support change. Williams and Walker (2003, p.134) report on how imagination can open up the 'possible options of behaving in future similar situations' and 'the possible outcomes if these different options were to be completed'. A core aspect of using imagination in a reflective group is using the group as a means of grounding imagined possibilities by discussing these and establishing their suitability. Whilst imagination and creativity can occur in one-to-one situations, there is a greater potential for these to flourish in group settings, where encouragement from other members of the group can help open up a creative streak that had previously been untapped. However, whilst some participants may find it relatively easy to access their creative side, others may find it more difficult to let go and think in a truly imaginative way. The facilitator needs to recognise this tension and support all members of the group to draw on their creativity and imagination. Many of the greatest inventions and innovations have arisen from people using their imagination and thinking innovatively. As a children's nurse, I often draw on children's literature as a basis for reflection and one of the Dr Seuss books is a great starting place. The book requires readers to think the unthinkable and to use their imagination. The final lines of the book *Oh, the Thinks You Can Think!* are a clarion call to think imaginatively and a good place to start a reflective group session, where the facilitator will be asking people to draw on their imagination:

'Think left and think right and think low and think high. Oh, the thinks you can think up if only you try!'

Power, groups and facilitation

An important difference between individual and group approaches is that group work takes reflection out of a relatively private domain between the two people involved and makes it a much more communal approach, as the reflection occurs between the members of the group (Fazio 2009). This shifts reflection from the private into a more public sphere of engagement.

Used thoughtlessly, group reflection can feel threatening (Bold 2008) and may create feelings of vulnerability (McGrath and Higgins 2006) and discomfort (Holmlund *et al.* 2010). The 'reflective contract' moves from being between two people to being between all members of the group. Everyone has to 'act well' for reflective group work to be really effective. Group work is most effective when the conditions are right. A crucial condition is the involvement of a skilled and experienced facilitator (Holmlund *et al.* 2010; Knight *et al.* 2010), whose role is to prepare participants, create a supportive environment, encourage engagement with the process and be vigilant for problems which might arise. The facilitator also needs to be aware that participants bring their previous experiences of reflection and group work; some of these experiences may be negative (Walsh *et al.* 2003).

Effective facilitation requires skilled facilitators who are confident and able to help the members negotiate challenging situations to ensure that they can gain the most from the reflective group sessions (Mastoras and Andrews 2011). Novice facilitators can find it difficult to elicit the best engagement from participants and often report finding managing group dynamics challenging (see, for example, McGrath and Higgins 2006). Gould and Masters (2004) note that the style of facilitation is crucial and that the role of the facilitator is demanding.

Although Bold (2008, p.265) notes the potential for peer support and 'mutual facilitation', the role of facilitator has most often been adopted by a senior person, either based within the practice setting or from an associated education setting. The drawback of this somewhat hierarchical-external-expert approach is that the reflective activity may become muddled with line management and be perceived more like surveillance than support (Stevenson 2005). Group participants often respond to such perceived risks by declining to engage and being selective about what they bring to the reflective group and this may sanitise the issues they reflect upon (Clouder and Sellars 2004). Whilst 'holding back' may be a

Chapter 4

mechanism employed by participants who perceive themselves as being less powerful and/or expert than the facilitator (or other group participants), in reality it can be a very effective, albeit subtle, means of exerting passive power over the group. Passive or active misuse/abuse of power is detrimental to group dynamics.

Some groups overcome potential power issues by making membership relatively homogeneous (similar grades or experiences). Other groups perceive that the potential richness in a diversity of experience and knowledge, that a more heterogeneous group can hold, outweighs any inherent risks. Diverse groups may generate and share greater insights into organisational culture and practice than one-to-one practices. This breadth of insight can give rise to extensive opportunities for genuine learning. Critical reflection (in a community of practice) can encourage professionals to address 'larger issues in ambiguous environments' (Ng and Tan 2009, p.41), ensuring that participants' reflection is not just inward looking.

Benefits of reflective group work

Many of the benefits of reflective groups arise from the dialogue that is an intrinsic element of their structure. The benefits of reflective group work include developing capacity and confidence, being supportive, helping to illuminate and enhance aspects of practice, improving the patient's/client's experience of care and problem solving (see, for example, Bold 2008; Fazio 2009; Severinsson et al. 2010). These benefits have potential for nurses throughout their careers. Reflective groups have been used effectively with students taking their first steps towards developing an understanding of their professional role (Gould and Masters 2004), as well as with experienced practitioners developing their leadership skills (Alleyne and Jumaa 2007) or strategic skills (Young et al. 2010) and taking on the challenges of driving nursing practice forward. Some studies, such as Ashmore et al. (2012), have suggested that group reflection may be perceived to be less threatening than individual reflection.

Lindahl and Norberg (2002, p.816) note that reflective group work with staff working in intensive care helped support them to manage 'professional and personally demanding complex nursing care'. The participants valued the cohesiveness that developed as a result of working within the group, which they felt could not have been developed in a one-to-one approach. Saarikoski et al. (2006, p.283) found that group reflection provided support to mental health nursing students who became less anxious about their ability to manage the 'unfamiliar emotional and psychological demands of practice'. In this same study, they also noted that group supervision was more positive in fostering a sense of professional identity than the one-to-one control group. Holm et al. (1998, p.109) found that process-oriented group supervision sessions, which aimed to help nursing students develop their nursing identity, had beneficial effects including 'sharing experiences of actions and reactions'. The students also 'learnt to listen more actively to each other and to achieve greater integration of their own and others' experiences of work'. In another study focusing on students, Holmlund *et al.* (2010, p.685) showed the growth that students could attain and noted that:

> 'By mirroring themselves in the eyes of the group members, the students could be provided with relief, confirmation and challenges. By listening to their peer students' narratives and viewpoints, their open-mindedness and empathy could be fostered'.

Certainly, personal experience supports the value of group-based reflection in terms of its value in identity development. Whilst facilitating a group of doctoral candidates from different academic disciplines and trying to encourage them to embrace the shift needed to perceive themselves as researchers and clinical academics, the value of different disciplinary perspectives was clear. As one participant reflected:

> 'It's curious really. I seem to be finding out more about who I am as a PhD student by listening to the guys from physics and computing. By hearing how they are facing some of the same challenges as I am it makes me feel that nursing is not so very different. It feels so hard sometimes to be doing a PhD whilst I'm working clinically. I don't know why I expect colleagues to understand as even I don't really know what a PhD is. What's clearer now is that all of us here are wanting to get our PhDs, not just because it means all the pain will stop but I think we want to be the person that the PhD will make us. That sounds tortuous but I'm changing … I think it's worth it … I know I think differently … I'm beginning to imagine that I will get there … not just to have a PhD but kind of be a PhD …'

Group supervision in Arvidsson *et al.*'s (2000, p.184–5) study focused on supporting psychiatric nurses to develop competence as professionals. The nurses in this study gained increased trust in their own performance, feelings and abilities and became 'more courageous, dared more and worked independently to a greater extent'. Over time, they felt they had greater trust in themselves and their competence as professionals. Similar outcomes in terms of professional and personal growth were evident in Severinsson *et al.*'s (2010) study where midwives who engaged in reflective group sessions felt that the reflection influenced their professional competence, as it supported them to integrate science into their practice whilst increasing their awareness of and sensitivity in their professional role. Central to this was 'an increased ability to reflect and greater creativity in practical situations' (Severinsson *et al.* 2010, p.405). An increase in participants' introspective ability was noted in Arillo *et al.*'s (2009) study of multiprofessional groups. Lecturers in Ashmore *et al.*'s (2012) study also

Chapter 4

felt that reflective group sessions promoted students' ability to reflect and solve problems, as well as helping them to understand their own personal strengths and weaknesses and ability to cope. It also enabled students to 'think creatively and to understand how to take responsibility for their own learning'.

In summary, therefore, although reflective groups can be risky, they can also be beneficial as they can assist participants to advance their own skills and knowledge whilst giving them the opportunity to draw on their own experiences to support their colleagues.

Challenges to group reflection

Whilst participants in group supervision will generally report positive aspects, group settings may cause anticipatory anxiety. This anxiety can be seen as one of the challenging aspects of group work since, if it is not managed effectively, it can stop a group from working well. Some anxiety is natural and to be expected (Walsh et al. 2003) but good facilitation can do a great deal to overcome this in the initial meetings (Ashmore et al. 2012).

Whilst facilitators and other stakeholders may be convinced of the value of reflective group working, these benefits may not be obvious to potential participants. Indeed, Knight et al.'s (2010) study showed that participants (trainee clinical psychologists) who were required to take part in reflective practice groups as part of their studies could be placed into one of two categories: those who saw the groups as valuable (n=74) and those who perceived the groups to result in high distress (n=45). Of the high distress group, 17 participants felt that the groups were also of low value to them. Reasons for this distress were related to group size (larger groups were more stressful), the style of facilitation (less robust facilitation increased distress) and being unclear about the group's purpose.

The level of distress reported in Knight et al.'s (2010) study seems a little atypical when compared with the anxiety reported in other studies. However, this may reflect the reporting tool, the fact that the participants were trainee clinical psychologists rather than nurses, or the choice of the word 'distress' rather than 'anxiety'. Studies fairly consistently report that reflective groups provoke anxiety (Lindgren et al. 2005; Jones 2006; McGrath and Higgins 2006; Knight et al. 2010). However, this anxiety is often reported to lessen as participants become accustomed to group membership. Personal experience, both as a group member and a facilitator of groups, reflects feelings of anxiety which generally subside as trust develops and clarity about the purpose of the group and insight into performance are gained. Lindgren et al. (2005), for example, note that in their study of group supervision of Swedish student nurses, 25% had negative expectations about group supervision before they commenced it. At the end of their group supervision programme, all the students felt that group supervision had been personally and professionally important and they wanted to continue to engage in group supervision after they had qualified. Interestingly, nearly half of the participants in Knight *et al.*'s (2010, p.435) study found it 'easier to see the value of the groups and appreciate the challenges in retrospect, after qualifying'.

Some nurses can be reticent about discussing sensitive or personal aspects of their practice. Jones (2006, p.161) states that hospice nurses 'found aspects of group work anxiety invoking and took time to trust and settle into the group task because of personal concerns … [*and that*] initial interactions suggested that psychological and social defences were preventing group members from sharing experiences openly'. Participants in group reflection can be anxious not only about what to share but also about whether or not they are approaching the reflection session correctly (McGrath and Higgins 2006). Reassurance about the process, expectations and ground rules can mitigate participants' concerns about whether they are doing things right.

Reticence can be evident in online groups as well as in face-to-face groups and it can be evident regardless of whether the engagement is with first-year pre-registration students, doctoral candidates and/or expert nurses. Indeed, experience suggests that groups composed of senior and expert nurses can create specific facilitation challenges. Expert participants tend to feel that they have more to lose and need to maintain a strong image within the group. As one participant explained during an early reflective group meeting for senior nurses:

> 'It's hard enough to just to be sat here, yet alone contemplating "spilling all" to people you don't know well. I spend most of my days in work, trying to be a role model, leading by example and yet in this room I'm expected to peel back some of my defences and talk reflectively about my practice. That feels almost impossibly hard at the moment. I can see the point of it. I like the sound of it. But I'm not sure I'm ready for it'.

This 'admission' opened a floodgate and the other participants showed their support and many of them confirmed that they were also feeling hesitant and anxious about the risks associated with sharing their experiences and feelings. One of the other participants summed this up by saying:

> 'Practice is often so demanding and draining and yet there's not many people you can turn to for support, people who you can trust. I don't feel I can talk to the people I manage about feeling angry about some things – that wouldn't be professional. And I certainly don't feel like I could talk to my line manager! So if things work out, this group could be absolutely brilliant for me – potentially a life and sanity saver'.

Over time, this group blossomed into a safe and supportive structure, a haven where participants shared difficulties they were facing, provided different perspectives and solutions, provided support for each other and reduced the feelings of isolation experienced in senior management.

Running a group: ground rules and other pragmatic issues

Running a reflective group, whether online or face to face, is challenging and there is no recipe for getting it right. However, there are a number of areas that anyone who is thinking of facilitating a group should consider. Box 4.2 provides an overview of core principles for facilitating group reflection and Box 4.3 provides an overview of the key processes/phases in facilitating a reflective group.

Box 4.2   Behaviours which will facilitate learning in group reflection (Developed from Mumford 1996, p.8)

- Ensuring everyone in the group a fair and appropriate share of the available time
- Being non-defensive about own actions and reflections
- Supporting the issues/concerns that group members raise
- Being open in initiating and responding to issues
- Being analytical and thoughtful about the reflections raised
- Adopting a challenging but constructive approach to eliciting further information
- Listening effectively
- Summarising accurately without undue interpretation
- Being creative, imaginative and solution oriented in response to identified challenges/problems
- Being insightful about the reflections that are being shared
- Being able to take risks and being aware that you are taking them and are aware of potential consequences
- Using strengths/resourcefulness of group members and not over-relying on own experiences/expertise
- Motivating and encouraging all members of the group and valuing individual contributions
- Supporting less vocal, less confident members of the group to share their experiences
- Praising people's efforts
- Providing direction as appropriate
- Developing ground rules with the group that are meaningful, contextualised and sustainable
- Knowing when to keep quiet – valuing silence.

Box 4.3   Overview of key processes/phases in facilitating a reflective group

Before the meeting	• The facilitator needs to find a comfortable venue that is conducive to reflective discussion. • Invite participants to the group, ensuring they know where the venue is. • Provide participants with information about the aims of the group. • Ensure that there is sufficient time for the first meeting.
At the start of the first meeting	• Create a safe and positive environment for the participants in the group in which they can work and share their ideas. • Use 'ice breakers' with the participants to help them get to know each other. This is also useful in a group where people know each other. These ice breaker activities need not be complicated but can involve asking questions about each other's areas of practice or something outside professional life such as where they went on their last holiday. Sharing this information with the group starts to provide some insight into their practice as well as revealing something about the participants as individuals. Taking notes can act as an effective *aide mémoire*. • Ensure that participants have an underpinning knowledge of the reflective process and how it will work within a group setting. • Assure participants that if they feel challenged and somewhat uncomfortable at times, this is not unusual and explore ways of dealing with this.
Develop the ground rules	• Every group will develop its own ground rules based on what is important to participants. However, some rules are fairly fundamental and seen in most reflective practice groups: confidentiality, listening, being non-judgemental, having the right to stay silent, and starting and ending the group on time.
Group discussion time	• Enable participants to contribute and recall events they wish to discuss. Ensure participants appreciate that they can share incidents of good practice as well as situations where they feel they did not do as well as they wanted to. • Analyse the issues using your chosen reflective model/framework. • Explore the theory–practice links. • Identify the lessons to learn from the incidents discussed. • Identify actions that can be taken to achieve the purpose of the group.

Contd.

At the end of the group	• Summarise the group activity.
	• Identify any actions that participants need to take in preparation for the next meeting and/or as a result of this meeting.
	• Thank everyone for their attendance.
	• Check that all the participants are OK, particularly if anyone appeared distressed, angry or very withdrawn.

Membership, micro-politics and the need to be accommodating

There is usually an unwritten tacit assumption that something as beneficial as membership of a reflective group is a personal choice. Yet for many participants there is little opportunity to decline membership or choose who they want to be in their group. Reflective groups are often instigated as a core element of a course or are an essential component of their work. Even when membership is not mandatory, declining to participate can be viewed as failing to engage and an indication that the individual is churlish, foolish or pig-headed. This pressure to participate is rarely acknowledged but this coercive drive means that many groups start with some 'members' who have been 'volunteered' or compelled to attend. It is a less than an auspicious start to a reflective group if a percentage of the people in the group feel resentful or angry.

Some groups have a fixed or closed membership whilst others may adopt a more fluid approach, allowing people to join and leave during the life of the group. Neither is the perfect approach and ultimately the choice is dependent on the reason(s) for the group forming, contextual factors, the degree of sensitivity of the issues to be discussed and, at a more pragmatic level, the practicalities involved. Groups where people are already known to each other, for example when they are made up of staff working in a particular team or setting, may benefit from that existing knowledge of each other. However, a limitation of this is that 'colleagues may hold similar views, restricting the extent to which any benefits of supervision are experienced by the team as whole' (Cleary and Freeman 2005, p.491). Whilst trust may develop more easily in a closed group, this should not be the primary reason for closed membership. In groups where participants work together outside the group setting, conflicts and tensions arising within the reflective sessions can be taken back into the workplace. Care needs to be taken by both the facilitator and the participants that any friction is 'parked' in the reflective group. Open groups, which necessarily have to be more flexible and accommodating, may more genuinely reflect everyday practice and the 'rivalries and micro-politics of the workplace' (Eraut 2004, p.49). Winship and Hardy (1999) concur that some of the conflicts and difficulties experienced in group work can prepare nurses for dealing with the sorts of conflicts that occur in clinical practice situations. They wryly note that even for the 'most inveterate of optimistic staff, there were times when the group was inescapably excruciating and difficult to bear as conflicts surfaced and harsh words were shared' (p.309). Holmlund *et al.* (2010) note that through reflective group work, students had learnt about the need to be honest and open-minded and they were able to create boundaries.

Group time and commitment to the group

Time is an important issue for reflective groups in terms of how many times a group meets, how frequently it meets, when it meets (time of day/night, day of the week) and how long it meets for. Some of this is determined by external factors such as the time pressures associated with the purpose of the group. For example, a reflective group may be tasked with completing their work within 6 months to fit in with external deadlines; other groups will be constrained by the reflection occurring during one specific module. Other resource constraints can be financial, as the number of meetings might be limited by the budget to support such meetings, or the amount of time an organisation is prepared to allow staff to be away from their core work. Time is less of an issue in online groups, particularly when based on asynchronous discussions. The final decisions are often pragmatic ones that try and ensure that attention is paid to best reflective group practice within the limitations and constraints imposed by the real world. However, these limitations can affect the outcomes of the group. As Saarikoski *et al.* (2006) reflect, their group of student nurses was less than cohesive, which they put down to the fact that they only met five times as a group during the course of a 5-week clinical placement.

The group also has to determine what level of priority the group activity is accorded, so that the time and space for the group are protected from other concerns. Protecting group time is important (Platzer 2004), as this is an essential prerequisite to ensuring that the group actually does happen, and that people within the group have an equitable opportunity to contribute. Walsh *et al.* (2002) note that their participants sometimes found it difficult to arrange times to meet due to clinical commitments, sick leave, annual leave and changes in the ward roster. However, commitment to the group is usually one of the ground rules that the group will set and aim to abide by. Asynchronous online groups can help overcome some of these problems but they still require commitment and engagement from participants.

Other ground rules usually focus on issues of confidentiality, respecting other people's opinions, not interrupting and preparing appropriately for the group. These rules are relatively easy to write and can be equally easy to commit to but it is often more difficult to consistently put them into practice. The dynamic nature of group discussion means that adhering to ground rules is anything but effortless; this in itself can be a good source of learning and reflection.

One core ground rule that does not always appear in textbooks is the need to start and end the group on time. This can be challenging for synchronous online groups whose members are from different time zones. Ensuring a timely finish may mean that the facilitator has to bring a lively discussion to a premature end. Successful facilitation of this can be achieved by acknowledging that the discussion is important, summarising and documenting the issues and assuring participants that any loose ends can be picked up at the next meeting or, where appropriate, arranging to meet up with individuals to discuss them between the scheduled group meetings.

Explaining the purpose of a reflective group

Ensuring that every member of a group (from the very enthusiastic to the more cynical and resistant) has a clear idea of the purpose of the group is absolutely crucial. Eraut (2004, p.49) reflects that often 'members of a group have very different agendas'. For example, drawing from personal experience of facilitating a group whose purpose was to discuss and decide upon a specific practice development, some members saw the group as a genuine opportunity to radically reconsider this aspect of practice, whilst others saw it as a means of identifying ways of reducing the number of trained nurses available to provide care. It took a while for the conspiracy theories to subside. Reflecting after the group, I noted in my journal:

> 'It's interesting … Whilst I was clarifying the purpose of the group and trying to provide reassurance that the outcomes of the group could be transformative to practice there was the start of a niggle that the conspiracy theorists might actually be right. I'm external to the group and to the setting and I feel a sense of doom about the thought that I could be responsible for the erosion of nursing in this setting … I need to think more … I guess as a nurse my first thoughts should always be for the patients but it's easy at times to want to defend practice … which gets muddled up and muddied up and it can easily mean focusing on protecting nurses and nursing rather than patient experiences …'

Ashmore *et al.* (2012, p.4) identified that some students 'struggled to orientate themselves to the purpose of the group'. This is fairly typical of many situations where students may have a very different understanding of the purpose of the group from the lecturer who is facilitating it. In some situations, there can be multiple groups and multiple facilitators; for example, where each of the wards and services in a clinical business unit is running its own reflective development groups to try and improve discharge planning, each facilitator needs to have a clear understanding of the purpose of the groups so that they can impart a clear and consistent message to their members. The facilitator has a key role in making the purpose explicit and transparent, as it can help the facilitator to effectively guide the group to maintain an appropriate focus. However, the participants also have a responsibility to develop their own insight into the purpose of the group, examine their assumptions and consider how they can contribute.

Eliciting reflections: dialogue and other approaches

One of the core tasks for a facilitator is to help the group maintain focus on the topic area, without having the lens so narrowly directed that opportunities to explore alternative options and ideas are missed. There needs to be a balance between staying on and going off message. The lecturers in Ashmore *et al.*'s (2012) study noted that the students needed help especially at the beginning of the course, to remain focused on their reflective tasks. Although Ashmore *et al.* proposed that the 'problem could potentially be avoided by the adoption of a more directive approach to supervision', they were less sure whether or not the facilitators would have welcomed this. Bold (2008, p.265) also noticed that many of the students in her study had difficulty in 'maintaining focus'.

Frequently, reflective groups are simply dialogue based and this is a sound approach to use. Group dialogue may be initiated by a question, a shared incident from practice, a news headline, an article or maybe the need to respond to a change in the workplace. However, sometimes it is helpful to use additional methods to prompt or sustain reflection.

Reflective journals and diaries (Chirema 2007; Leeuwen *et al.* 2009; Bedwell *et al.* 2012; Mabbett *et al.* 2011), reflective blogs (Killeavy and Moloney 2010) and other forms of 'blended learning' (Rigby *et al.* 2012) can all be used to support participants to prepare for and take action consequent to reflective groups or, in the case of reflective blogs, by sustaining reflection and connection between participants between group meetings.

Asking people to think imaginatively, using an arts- or activities-based approach, can be liberating for participants. The choice of which activity to use is largely dependent on the confidence of the facilitator and the flexibility of the group, as well as pragmatic issues such as the location and timing of the group. Activities which can stimulate overtly imaginative and creative thinking can include collage, drawing, drama, quilting, as well as perhaps simpler approaches such as getting people to write postcards to an appropriately influential person in which, for example, they outline what they imagine their service could look like if changes were made. Arts-based approaches can sometimes be resisted by participants who feel that they are a distraction from the main work of the group. However, from personal experience as both facilitator and group member, arts-based approaches can be both surprisingly powerful and hugely enjoyable, and it is good for people to appreciate

Chapter 4

that serious outcomes can be achieved whilst having fun. This in itself is often a good point to reflect upon.

The need to challenge, the need to support

It is clear that reflective groups are not an easy option but the rewards can be commensurately large. Challenge is intrinsic to reflection and it is only through exploring the conflict and contradictions that arise within reflection that participants can move beyond habitual responses (McGill and Beaty 2001). Bold (2008, p.265) notes that reflection in peer support groups provided participants with the 'opportunity to review memories of events, replay them through discussion and to rethink current practice'. Interestingly, Walsh *et al.* (2003, p.39) note that community nurses compromised their 'ability to reflect upon and critique practice' because in their 'effort to be supportive they did not sufficiently challenge each other'.

Developing a supportive environment does not just happen; it requires active effort from all the participants, it builds over time and some risks have to be taken. Each group will create and sustain their own supportive environment, because it is dependent on the experiences, expectations and commitments of the individuals within the group. Holmlund *et al.* (2010, p.685) note that students had positive experiences in 'stable groups of equals, in which they felt safe, were taken seriously and were listened to'. As a group develops a sense of safety, boundaries can be pushed and from personal experience this is the point at which reflection can really start to fly and some of the exciting, edgy and innovative outcomes can be achieved.

One of the challenges of group work is ensuring that every participant is engaged within the group. An appropriate amount of time needs to be available so that reflection can occur in sufficient depth, and that, over an agreed period of time, everyone's stories and experiences are shared and addressed appropriately. Poor time management can sometimes lead to even the initially enthusiastic group members disengaging from the process. It is equally important to ensure that no one individual or 'faction' monopolises the group. Lindahl and Norberg (2002, p.816) identified that time constraints with the groups they were researching hindered 'deep narratives'. Group size and time constraints mean that every group has to work within limits on the length and detail of the narratives that can be shared. Whilst in a large group the facilitator might try to ensure that every participant is able to say something in every session, this might not be the best use of time. Short superficial presentations constrain the quality and depth of any reflection (Eraut 2004).

Engagement should be considered across the life of the group. If some participants are initially reluctant to contribute, then although the facilitator should provide openings for their engagement, personal experience suggests that being pushy is counterproductive. Engagement is generally seen in terms of contributing verbally (or via text in online groups). However, contributions can be more subtle and may initially be through body language, for example through leaning forward, nodding and so on. Giving participants the space to take their time with contributions is valuable.

In one reflective group I was facilitating which was composed of parents of children with disabilities and the health professionals who provided services to them, one of the parents took several sessions to contribute. I was aware of his silence but was also aware that the group seemed fine with this. He was not unfriendly or aloof and during the tea and coffee at the start of the group he joined in the general conversation. It seemed to me that he was biding his time and at the time I was using a fair amount of facilitative energy in trying to rein in one of the more voluble members of the group. However, the quiet parent interjected into the other participants' stream of consciousness and said:

> 'I'm sorry to interrupt but I think the problem is that that's a good argument but you're completely missing the point. It's not what you want as a service that's important to me and my child, it's more of a case of what my child needs should be shaping your service. At least that's what I think ….'

The impact on the group was extraordinary and well worth the wait of several weeks. The more voluble member of the group was visibly moved and as she described later in the session:

> 'I felt G [*the quiet parent*] kind of rebooted my hard drive. I felt like that what he said was so important and it's not that I didn't really know what he said was true. It was more that I didn't feel it until he said it in this group. Like I say it feels like my head has got a new operating system installed – newer and better and more focused on the children and families … that's got to be good'.

Whilst there are no hard and fast rules about group size, it is important to consider the effects that group size has on group dynamics (Knight *et al.* 2010) and the ability to reflect in depth. Groups with around eight members have a good chance of functioning well; relationships can be developed and sharing of deep narratives can occur and participants generally do not feel too fazed by contributing within a group of this size.

Reflecting on people and situations

Due care needs to be taken when discussing other people and their lives; this is regardless of whether they are patients/clients, their relatives, colleagues, friends or family. Anonymity should be maintained. Group members need to listen attentively so that they will be able to contribute thoughtfully to the reflective discussion arising from the shared incident.

Recalling and sharing an incident lays the person who is relating the incident open to the scrutiny and judgement of others. Apart from rare incidents where it is clear that someone was acting unprofessionally, it is important that participants respect the decisions made by other people and understand that the actions they took occurred in a particular setting and context. This does not mean to say that the actions taken and responses to these actions cannot be reflected upon and practice improved in some way. Of course, any unprofessional activity would need to be followed up and appropriate action taken in line with the Nursing and Midwifery Council's Code of Conduct (Nursing and Midwifery Council 2008). Careful judgement needs to be taken on how any actions taken are reported back to the group.

Facilitation and 'flying solo'

Pedler and Abbott (2008) talk of facilitators adopting the role of initiator, leader and coach, and whilst they talk of these in terms of action learning sets, these roles have resonance within many reflective group settings. Many groups will draw upon the skills of a facilitator in their early stages, although in most cases facilitators should be working towards assisting the group to become self-facilitating (see, for example, Holmes 2008). Otherwise, paradoxically, a group that is reflecting on issues such as empowerment, independence and autonomy could remain dependent and disempowered. This approach is particularly true for action learning sets where part of the facilitator's role is to model effective styles and approaches to questions and communication (McGill and Beaty 2001). Setting a reflective group free of their facilitator is not always achieved, as was apparent in Stark's (2006) study. She notes that where educators regularly attended set meetings, they quickly learnt processes which were effective in helping the group take over facilitation. However, in the sets where attendance was more erratic, they needed more sustained facilitation to keep the projects moving forward (Stark 2006, p.27).

Supporting facilitators

Facilitators need supervision (Rolfe *et al.* 2001; Ashmore *et al.* 2012). Facilitating a group is not an easy role and it demands an ethical and moral response from the facilitator. Agelii *et al.* (2000, p.358), in their study of the ethical dimensions of group supervision, conclude that one of the responsibilities of the supervisor/facilitator is 'to create a moral reflective mental space'. It requires skill to help participants make their own decisions and come to their conclusions concerning incidents from practice. Given that the incidents chosen for discussion may be distressing, facilitators may find themselves on something of an emotional rollercoaster. From personal experience this can be draining, demanding and difficult.

Interestingly, whilst supervision is seen as being an important tool in dealing with the vicarious distress and trauma that can be encountered in practice (Bell *et al.* 2003; Jones and Cutcliffe 2009), there is much less written about how the facilitator should deal with their own distress that may arise as a result of listening to a series of traumatic incidents. Even less acknowledgement has been given to possible group distress and how to deal with it. At the very least, the facilitator needs to be aware of the potential of being overwhelmed by difficult stories and take care that they have access to support for their own emotional and professional needs. Writing a reflective journal has been profoundly supportive for me in helping me to regain equilibrium and develop greater insights into what was going on, how I could have handled things better, and whether the distress had been a useful part of the reflection process.

Conclusion: many hands or too many cooks?

Within this chapter, the nature of group reflection has been explored. Since groups are likely to be 'here to stay', it is important to acknowledge the benefits which can accrue as a result of the particular dynamics and resonances which can develop between members of a group. However, it is also important to note that group reflection is complex and challenging. The adage that 'many hands make light work' can be true within group reflection; the range of perspectives that can be shared can illuminate problems and provide a breadth and depth of resource that is difficult to match in a one-to-one setting. However, another adage comes to mind: 'too many cooks spoil the broth'. Ineffective group work can arise from a number of factors, including poorly managed contributions from partici-pants, active and passive resistance to the group and a lack of focus.

Reflective group work is powerful and fragile. It has enormous potential but it requires commitment and courage from the participants and the ability to create a safe and secure environment from the facilitator. Reflective groups have the potential to help nurses change their worlds. Ghaye (2008, p.1) suggests that reflective practice should be thought of 'more as a political and collective process and not only as a professional and individualistic practice'. With this approach to reflecting in groups, nurses can surely try to live up to Mead's challenge with which I opened the chapter, that within small groups we can change the world.

References

Abma, T.A. (2007) Situated learning in communities of practice: evaluation of coercion in psychiatry as a case. *Evaluation*, **13**, 32–47.

Agélii, E., Kennergren, B., Severinsson, E. and Berthold, H. (2000) Ethical dimen-sions of supervision: the supervisors' experiences. *Nursing Ethics*, **7**, 350–359.

Alleyne, J.O. and Jumaa, M.O. (2007) Building the capacity for evidence-based clinical nursing leadership: the role of executive co-coaching and group clinical supervision for quality patient services. *Journal of Nursing Management*, **15**, 230–243.

Arillo, C.A., Zabalegui Ardaiz, M.J., Ayarra, E.M., Fuertes, G.C., Loayssa Lara, J.R. and Pascual, P.P. (2009) [The reflection group as a tool for improving satisfaction and developing the introspective ability of health professionals]. *Aten Primaria*, **41**, 688–694.

Arvidsson, B., Lofgren, H. and Fridlund, B. (2000) Psychiatric nurses' conceptions of how group supervision in nursing care influences their professional competence. *Journal of Nursing Management*, **8**, 175–185.

Ashmore, R., Carver, N., Clibbens, N. and Sheldon, J. (2012) Lecturers' accounts of facilitating clinical supervision groups within a pre-registration mental health nursing curriculum. *Nurse Education Today*, **32**(3), 224–228.

Bedwell, C., McGowan, L. and Lavender, T. (2012) Using diaries to explore midwives' experiences in intrapartum care: an evaluation of the method in a phenomenological study. *Midwifery*, **28**(2), 150–155.

Bell, H., Kulkarni, S. and Dalton, L. (2003) Organizational prevention of vicarious trauma. *Families in Society: The Journal of Contemporary Human Services*, **84**, 463–474.

Berry, L.E. (2011) Creating community: strengthening education and practice partnerships through communities of practice. *International Journal of Nursing Education Scholarship*, **8**, 1–18.

Bold, C. (2008) Peer support groups: fostering a deeper approach to learning through critical reflection on practice. *Reflective Practice*, **9**, 257–267.

Booth, A., Sutton, A. and Falzon, L. (2003) Working together: supporting projects through action learning. *Health Information and Libraries Journal*, **20**, 225–231.

Burton, J. (2004) *Understanding and Promoting Work Based Learning in Primary Care*, 2nd edn. Radcliffe Medical Press, Oxford, pp.199–201.

Buus, N., Angel, S., Traynor, M. and Gonge, H. (2011) Psychiatric nursing staff members' reflections on participating in group-based clinical supervision: a semistructured interview study. *International Journal of Mental Health Nursing*, **20**, 95–101.

Cassidy, L. (2011) Online communities of practice to support collaborative mental health practice in rural areas. *Issues in Mental Health Nursing*, **32**, 98–107.

Chirema, K.D. (2007) The use of reflective journals in the promotion of reflection and learning in post-registration nursing students. *Nurse Education Today*, **27**, 192–202.

Cleary, M. and Freeman, A. (2005) The cultural realities of clinical supervision in an acute inpatient mental health setting. *Issues in Mental Health Nursing*, **26**, 489–505.

Clouder, L. and Sellars, J. (2004) Reflective practice and clinical supervision: an interprofessional perspective. *Journal of Advanced Nursing*, **46**, 262–269.

Dealey, C., Moss, H., Marshall, J. and Elcoat, C. (2007) Auditing the impact of implementing the Modern Matron role in an acute teaching trust. *Journal of Nursing Management*, **15**, 22–33.

Dewar, B.J. and Walker, E. (1999) Experiential learning: issues for supervision. *Journal of Advanced Nursing*, **30**, 1459–1467.

Douglas, S. and Machin, T. (2004) A model for setting up interdisciplinary collaborative working in groups: lessons from an experience of action learning. *Journal of Psychiatric and Mental Health Nursing*, **11**, 189–193.

Ekebergh, M. (2011) A learning model for nursing students during clinical studies. *Nurse Education in Practice*, **11**, 384–389.

Eraut, M. (2004) *The Practice of Reflection*, 3rd edn. Blackwell Publishing, Oxford, pp.47–52.

Fazio, X. (2009) Teacher development using group discussion and reflection. *Reflective Practice*, **10**, 529–541.

Flanagan, J., Baldwin, S. and Clarke, D. (2000) Work-based learning as a means of developing and assessing nursing competence. *Journal of Clinical Nursing*, **9**, 360–368.

Garbett, R., Hardy, S., Manley, K., Titchen, A. and McCormack, B. (2007) Developing a qualitative approach to 360-degree feedback to aid understanding and development of clinical expertise. *Journal of Nursing Management*, **15**, 342–347.

Ghaye, T. (2008) *Building the Reflective Healthcare Organisation*. Wiley, Chichester.

Gherardi, S. (2001) From organizational learning to practice-based knowing. *Human Relations*, **54**, 131–139.

Gherardi, S. (2003) Knowing as desiring. Mythic knowledge and the knowledge journey in communities of practitioners. *Journal of Workplace Learning*, **15**, 352–358.

Gould, B. and Masters, H. (2004) Learning to make sense: the use of critical incident analysis in facilitated reflective groups of mental health student nurses. *Learning in Health and Social Care*, **3**, 53–63.

Hanson, K. (2011) 'Reflect' – is this too much to ask? *Reflective Practice*, **12**, 293–304.

Hardacre, J.E. and Keep, J. (2003) From intent to impact: developing clinical leaders for service improvement. *Learning in Health and Social Care*, **2**, 169–176.

Hardy, S., Titchen, A. and Manley, K. (2007) Patient narratives in the investigation and development of nursing practice expertise: a potential for transformation. *Nursing Inquiry*, **14**, 80–88.

Heiskanen, T. (2007) A knowledge-building community for public sector professionals. *Journal of Workplace Learning*, **16**, 370–384.

Hewison, A., Badger, F. and Swani, T. (2011) Leading end-of-life care: an action learning set approach in nursing homes. *International Journal of Palliative Nursing*, **17**, 135–141.

Holm, A., Lantz, I. and Severinsson, E. (1998) Nursing students' experiences of the effects of continual process-oriented group supervision. *Journal of Nursing Management*, **6**, 105–113.

Holmes, M. (2008) What do set facilitators bring to the party? (And do we need them?) *Action Learning: Research and Practice*, **5**, 249–253.

Holmlund, H., Lindgren, B. and Athlin, E.Y. (2010) Group supervision for nursing students during their clinical placements: its content and meaning. *Journal of Nursing Management*, **18**, 678–688.

Jones, A. (2003) Some benefits experienced by hospice nurses from group clinical supervision. *European Journal of Cancer Care*, **12**, 224–232.

Jones, A. (2006) Group-format clinical supervision for hospice nurses. *European Journal of Cancer Care*, **15**, 155–162.

Jones, A.C. and Cutcliffe, J.R. (2009) Listening as a method of addressing psychological distress. *Journal of Nursing Management*, **17**, 352–358.

Chapter 4

Kilcullen. N/ (2007) An analysis of the experiences of clinical supervision on Registered Nurses undertaking MSc/graduate diploma in renal and urological nursing and on their clinical supervisors. *Journal of Clinical Nursing*, **16**, 1029–1038.

Killeavy, M. and Moloney, A. (2010) Reflection in a social space: can blogging support reflective practice for beginning teachers? *Teaching and Teacher Education*, **26**, 1070–1076.

Knight, K., Sperlinger, D. and Maltby, M. (2010) Exploring the personal and professional impact of reflective practice groups: a survey of 18 cohorts from a UK clinical psychology training course. *Clinical Psychology and Psychotherapy*, **17**, 427–437.

Lathlean, J. and Le May, A. (2002) Communities of practice: an opportunity for interagency working. *Journal of Clinical Nursing*, **11**, 394–398.

Lee-Baldwin, J. (2005) Asynchronous discussion forums: a closer look at the structure, focus and group dynamics that facilitate reflective thinking. *Contemporary Issues in Technology and Teacher Education*, **5**, 93–115.

Leeuwen, R., Tiesinga, L.J., Jochemsen, H. and Post, D. (2009) Learning effects of thematic peer review: a qualitative analysis of reflective journals on spiritual care. *Nurse Education Today*, **29**, 413–422.

Lindahl, B. and Norberg, A. (2002) Clinical group supervision in an intensive care unit: a space for relief, and for sharing emotions and experiences of care. *Journal of Clinical Nursing*, **11**, 809–818.

Lindgren, B., Brulin, C., Holmlund, K. and Athlin, E. (2005) Nursing students' perception of group supervision during clinical training. *Journal of Clinical Nursing*, **14**, 822–829.

Mabbett, G.M., Jenkins, E.R., Surridge, A.G., Warring, J. and Gwynn, E.D. (2011) Supporting and supervising district nurse students through patchwork text writing. *Nurse Education in Practice*, **11**, 6–13.

Maggs, C. and Biley, A. (2000) Reflections on the role of the nursing development facilitator in clinical supervision and reflective practice. *International Journal of Nursing Practice*, **6**, 192–195.

Mann, K.V., Mcfetridge-Durdle, J., Martin-Misener, R., *et al.* (2009) Interprofessional education for students of the health professions: the 'Seamless Care' model. *Journal of Interprofessional Care*, **23**, 224–233.

Mastoras, S.M., Andrews, J.J.W. (2011) The supervisee experience of group supervision: implications for research and practice. *Training and Education in Professional Psychology*, **5**, 102–111.

McGill, I. and Beaty, L. (2001) *Action Learning: A Guide for Professional, Management and Educational Development*, 2nd edn. Taylor and Francis, Abingdon.

McGrath, D. and Higgins, A. (2006) Implementing and evaluating reflective practice group sessions. *Nurse Education in Practice*, **6**, 175–181.

Mumford, A. (1996) Effective learners in action learning sets. *Journal of Workplace Learning*, **8**, 3–10.

Ng, P.T. and Tan, C. (2009) Community of practice for teachers: sensemaking or critical reflective learning? *Reflective Practice*, **10**, 37–44.

Nursing and Midwifery Council (2008) *The Code. Standards of Conduct, Performance and Ethics for nurses and midwives.* Nursing and Midwifery Council, London.

O'Connell, B., Ockerby, C.M., Johnson, S., Smenda, H. and Bucknall, T.K. (2011) Team clinical supervision in acute hospital wards: a feasibility study. *Western Journal of Nursing Research* April 29 (Epub ahead of print).

O'Connor, N. and Kotze, B. (2008) 'Learning organizations': a clinician's primer. *Australasian Psychiatry*, **16**, 173–178.

Pedler, M. and Abbott, C. (2008) Am I doing it right? Facilitating action learning for service improvement. *Leadership in Health Services*, **21**, 185–199.

Platzer, H. (2004) Are you sitting uncomfortably? From group resistance to group reflection in several uneasy moves. In: Bulman, C. and Schutz, S. (eds) Reflective Practice in Nursing, 3rd edn. Blackwell Publishing, Oxford, pp.113–127.

Rigby, L., Wilson, I., Baker, J., *et al.* (2012) The development and evaluation of a 'blended' enquiry based learning model for mental health nursing students: 'making your experience count'. *Nurse Education Today*, **32**(3), 303–308.

Rivas, K. and Murray, S. (2010) Exemplar: our shared experience of implementing action learning sets in an acute clinical nursing setting: approach taken and lessons learned. *Contemporary Nurse: A Journal for the Australian Nursing Profession*, **35**, 182–187.

Rocco, S. (2010) Making reflection public: using interactive online discussion board to enhance student learning. *Reflective Practice*, **11**, 307–317.

Rolfe, G., Freshwater, D. and Jasper, M. (2001) Critical Reflection for Nursing and the Helping Professions: A User's Guide. Palgrave, Basingstoke.

Saarikoski, M., Warne, T., Aunio, R. and Leino-Kilpi, H. (2006) Group supervision in facilitating learning and teaching in mental health clinical placements: a case example of one student group. *Issues in Mental Health Nursing*, **27**, 273–285.

Severinsson, E., Haruna, M. and Friberg, F. (2010) Midwives' group supervision and the influence of their continuity of care model – a pilot study. *Journal of Nursing Management*, **18**, 400–408.

Shanley, M.J. and Stevenson, C. (2006) Clinical supervision revisited. *Journal of Nursing Management*, **14**, 586–592.

Sheehan, D. (2011) Clinical learning within a community of practice framework. *Focus on Health Professional Education: A Multi-disciplinary Journal*, **12**, 1.

Stark, S. (2006) Using action learning for professional development. *Educational Action Research*, **14**, 23–43.

Stevenson, C. (2005) Postmodernising clinical supervision in nursing. *Issues in Mental Health Nursing*, **26**, 519–529.

Walsh, K., McAllister, M. and Morgan, A. (2002) Using reflective practice processes to identify practice change issues in an aged care service. *Nurse Education in Practice*, **2**, 230–236.

Walsh, K., Nicholson, J., Keough, C., Pridham, R., Kramer, M. and Jeffrey, J. (2003) Development of a group model of clinical supervision to meet the needs of a community mental health nursing team. *International Journal of Nursing Practice*, **9**, 33–39.

Wenger, E. (2000) Communities of practice and social learning systems. *Organization*, **7**, 225.

White, E. and Winstanley, J. (2006) Cost and resource implications of clinical supervision in nursing: an Australian perspective. *Journal of Nursing Management*, **14**, 628–636.

Chapter 4

Williams, B. and Walker, L. (2003) Facilitating perception and imagination in generating change through reflective practice groups. *Nurse Education Today*, **23**, 131–137.

Williams, C. (2010) Understanding the essential elements of work-based learning and its relevance to everyday clinical practice. *Journal of Nursing Management*, **18**, 624–632.

Winship, G. and Hardy, S. (1999) Disentangling dynamics: group sensitivity and supervision. *Journal of Psychiatric and Mental Health Nursing*, **6**, 307–312.

Young, S., Nixon, E., Hinge, D., *et al.* (2010) Action learning: a tool for the development of strategic skills for nurse consultants? *Journal of Nursing Management*, **18**, 105–110.

Chapter 5

An exploration of the student and mentor journey into reflective practice

Charlotte Maddison and Pam Sharp

Faculty of Health and Life Sciences, Oxford Brookes University, Oxford, UK

Introduction

This chapter will outline the importance and relevance of reflection for both the student and mentor. It will briefly identify the key changes that are affecting professional practice and education. We will revisit the student and mentor journey into reflection and identify new developments and insights we have gained, plus we will consider again the skills needed for reflection. We will explore both the value and practical application of reflection in the university setting, in placement and in the simulated environment. For mentors, we will offer trigger questions for reflection on their role based on the Nursing and Midwifery Council (2008a) Standards to support learning and assessment in practice. Throughout this chapter we will provide examples taken from work with pre-registration students and their mentors, although some of the areas of discussion equate equally to those in postqualifying education.

Changes and pressures on nursing and education – why reflection is increasingly important for students and mentors

It will come as no surprise to those of you in practice or education when we assert that health and social care, including nursing, is in a state of constant change. The Royal College of Nursing (2011) commissioned a survey of 2000 nurses across the UK and outlined some of the ongoing issues affecting nurses including a challenging economic climate, increased numbers of patients with long-term conditions and ageing of the population.

Reflective Practice in Nursing, Fifth Edition. Edited by Chris Bulman and Sue Schutz.
© 2013 John Wiley & Sons, Ltd. Published 2013 by John Wiley & Sons, Ltd.

The survey highlighted that nurses are under increased pressure, with many stating that they were unable to deliver the standard of care they would like to, that safety was compromised, and that staffing levels were too low. Countries worldwide are experiencing the effect of financial constraints and this can affect actual numbers of nurses in the workplace and also changes in skill mix. For example, in the UK there is concern that government cuts are impacting negatively on UK nursing numbers (Triggle and Hughes 2011). These pressures may inevitably influence the number of available mentors. This in turn may then impact on opportunities for reflective activities between mentor and student.

Wilson (2010), a PhD student and lecturer, has discussed the demands on nurse mentors. The online discussion that followed her article indicates that there are strong feelings about the pressures facing those in the role of supporting students and that this affects both support and assessment roles. Both Magnusson et al. (2007) and Mallik and McGowan (2007) have previously reported on this ongoing issue and Mamede and Schmidt (2005) have noted that one of the barriers to reflection is time pressures. Similarly, Gopee (2011) has discussed the place of reflection in learning from experience, asserting that time should be made available after practice placements for reflection, consolidation and evaluation of learning to take place. The opportunity to do this may vary with the placement and shift patterns, and so this is where mentors need to act in a leadership role to negotiate and organise the time for reflection with their students.

Many countries are experiencing ageing populations and this means that nurses in all specialties may be caring for patients/clients with multiple pathologies and diverse care needs. These patients are likely to be more dependent and require increased time to carry out personalised and individual care. Where nurses make care decisions in these complex and unpredictable settings, reflection can play a key part in helping them to make sense of their practice and consider its effects (Teekman 2000). For example, if a nurse has been involved in making care decisions regarding a patient with multiple problems, they may want to fully reflect on the factors that influenced that decision making, consider what was good and bad about the process and outcome, in order to learn from it and apply that learning to future situations.

Reflection is a key component of clinical judgement, decision making, accountability and critical thinking. We believe that as students progress towards becoming professionals and develop their clinical judgement, they need to be able to reflect on the effectiveness of their decisions and on their practice. This needs to continue once nurses and midwives become qualified accountable professionals. The Nursing and Midwifery Council (2009, p.1) states that accountability is 'integral to professional practice' and as part of this, it describes clinical judgement as being where:

'Nurses and midwives use their professional knowledge, judgement and skills to make a decision based on evidence for best practice and the person's best interests. Nurses and midwives need to be able to justify the decisions they make'.

In the UK nurses and midwives are also obligated to adhere to the Code (Nursing and Midwifery Council 2008b, p.5) where it outlines that they should: 'Deliver care based on the best available evidence or best practice' and 'must take part in appropriate learning and practice activities' (Nursing and Midwifery Council 2008b, p.6).

Reflection can meet this need for a flexible learning activity. If nurses reflect on their day-to-day practice they are much more likely to be open to change, learn from their experiences and develop personally and professionally.

On top of this responsibility for their own development, the Code states that nurses and midwives have a responsibility to facilitate the learning of others, including students. Reflection and reflective activities can play a significant part in helping facilitate the learning of others too. It is hard not to see similarities between the skills and purposes of reflection and critical thinking (Aveyard *et al.* 2011). Indeed, Facione (2011, p.12) describes how 'critical thinking is purposeful, *reflective judgement* that is focused on deciding what to believe or what to do'. Therefore, as both students and professionals rise to the challenges and pressures outlined above, reflection is now, and will be, even more vital for effective clinical judgement, good decision making and self-aware practice.

The student's journey into reflection

How we introduce reflection to our students

The concept of reflection is introduced during the students' first practice-related module. This occurs in their initial semester and prepares them for their first placement experience. Fundamental skills and theoretical concepts are introduced and reflection is incorporated into all aspects of this taught module. This is first achieved by way of a lecture introducing reflective practice. Within this lecture, we ask students to consider knowledge and how nurses acquire it. This may at first be a difficult concept for students to grasp. However, with prompting, students usually identify the internet, books, journals and their mentors as sources of knowledge. We then challenge students to consider where their mentors acquire their own knowledge. This enables us to discuss Schön's (1987) concepts of the swampy lowlands and technical rationality of professional knowledge. Students learn that technical or scientific knowledge can easily provide the evidence for activities such as monitoring temperature for signs of infection, whereas other less clear-cut areas of knowledge exist. As discussed above, there are increased numbers of patients with complex needs, care may need to be delivered in busy, pressured environments and there may be decisions that cannot be helped by

Box 5.1   Types of nursing knowledge

Mantzoukas and Jasper (2008) investigated the types of knowledge that nurses employ in order to care for patients in hospital and found five types.

1. **Personal practice knowledge**: that is acquired during a meeting with a particular patient.
2. **Theoretical knowledge**: which is acquired through formal education.
3. **Procedural knowledge**: that relates to pattern recognition. It describes practice that relies on previous experience. The nurses were able to draw upon previous actions or observations and essentially replicate them. This type of knowledge is described in previous literature as inductive reasoning (Higgs and Jones 2000).
4. **Ward cultural knowledge**: which relates to the well-known customs and practices of the ward.
5. **Reflexive knowledge**: which is related to the synthesis of the four previous types of knowledge. Mantzoukas and Jasper observed that when faced with a similar situation, junior and senior nurses would often respond differently. They concluded that the junior nurse lacked the reflexive knowledge of the senior nurse. Reflexive knowledge is dependent on prior experience. Reflection upon experience is needed to enable junior nurses to increase their existing knowledge and affect future practice.

scientific knowledge alone. For example, how did a mentor know how to respond when a patient refused to have a wound dressing changed? This is the type of knowledge that is derived from experience and reflecting on that experience.

Both the work of Schön (1983) and Mantzoukas and Jasper (2008) (see Box 5.1) can help students to realise that learning does not just happen by default. It is an active process and involves a variety of experiences and situations. Students begin to understand that practice is not always straightforward and that reflection will assist them in making sense of experiences that are often stressful and complex. Students learn that in order to gain from a practice experience, they will benefit from critically analysing the situation and applying their newly gained perspective to future experiences.

Once this idea is understood, we introduce students to reflective frameworks, with Gibbs (1988) as the framework of choice because it derives from Kolb's (1984) principle of experiential learning, which is essentially how we want the students to learn. Students are also directed to a number of alternative frameworks such as Driscoll (2007) and then asked to choose the one that is most useful to them (see Chapter 9 for these and other frameworks). The overall aim of this first lecture is to make students aware that reflection can develop personal understanding, improve professional practice, develop care for clients, challenge attitudes and beliefs and aid clinical decision making. Having explored the process of reflection during this lecture, students then apply the principles during subsequent seminars, clinical skills sessions and placements. This allows them to more easily make links between theory and practice (O'Regan and Fawcett 2006).

Jasper (2006) noted that reflection can be used as a strategy which involves thinking about practice experiences, in order to help develop understanding and so inform practice. She outlined three stages of reflective practice:

1. experience
2. reflection
3. action.

The ultimate aim is to help students learn from that initial experience through reflection, which will then influence their actual performance as practitioners. Mann *et al.* (2009), in a systematic review exploring reflection and reflective practice in health professions education, identified that reflection is a useful tool that enables learners to integrate new knowledge with existing knowledge. However, they also recognised that the way in which reflection can contribute to learning is not always obvious to students and that to experienced qualified practitioners it may be 'a tacit process' (Mann *et al.* 2009, p.614), meaning that knowledge is intuitively embedded in practice and cannot always be easily explained. Therefore, the concept and process of reflection need to be explicitly incorporated into an education programme. This can be achieved by using Jasper's framework above.

Preparation for nursing practice in pre-registration programmes occurs through a variety of means and students will learn about nursing by engaging in different learning activities. These may involve role-play, discussion around case studies, simulated activities in the skills laboratory and experience in practice. Both Jasper (2006) and Fowler (2008) undertook an exploration of the literature and discussed the concept of experience-based learning. They acknowledged previous work (Kolb 1984) and suggested that learning will only take place if both an experience and an opportunity to reflect are present. Irrespective of the delivery method, the student will achieve the greatest learning if they are able to reflect upon the educational activity. This is particularly relevant to the learning that takes place in placement; however, students often require guidance and support when reflecting on practice so placing emphasis on the skill of mentors and academic staff in facilitating reflective activities is essential (Morris and Stew 2007).

Whilst a great amount of time is invested in preparing students to reflect upon their practice, success is often dependent upon the continuing support received in practice. Mentors will obviously play a key role; however, as discussed above, organisational and political pressures may impede this. Therefore the academic team can facilitate links between theory and practice by promoting reflection during contact meetings in the practice setting. What is clear is that students seem to benefit from being able to reflect upon experiences (O'Donovan 2005; Bulman 2008; Matthew and Sternberg 2009). Therefore it needs to be integrated throughout both the taught and practice parts of the programme and students require preparation in order to utilise the skills successfully. The Royal College of Nursing (2006) guide *Helping Students Get the Best from Their Practice Placements* continues to be a useful starting point for students and mentors in preparing for placement. It specifically asks that students reflect upon practice and that mentors facilitate reflection. We therefore encourage students and mentors to utilise it when planning placement activities.

Whilst we aim to instil in students all the skills for reflection, we recognise that this is a developmental process. In preparing students for their initial placements, we focus on the introduction of self-awareness.

Developing self-awareness in practice and the simulated environment

We believe that the concept of self-awareness is fundamental to nursing practice and is a required skill for reflection. Eckroth-Bucher (2010, p.308) concluded in a concept analysis of self-awareness that it is integral to 'creating an interpersonal environment that heals'. However, Eckroth-Bucher found that there is a lack of clarity or definition of self-awareness within the literature and that the meanings of self-awareness and reflection often overlap. Overall self-awareness can be identified not as an isolated component of reflection but a: 'dynamic, introspective, interweaving, process of thoughts, values, convictions, emotions, experience and feedback' (Eckroth-Bucher 2010, p.308).

Harrison and Fopma-Loy (2010) make reference to the concept of emotional intelligence, which requires a student to develop an understanding of themselves and how their actions will affect another. Despite the consensus that students should demonstrate emotional insight, Harrison and Fopma-Loy have suggested that increasingly nursing students show a 'disconnection' from the humanistic element of nursing, focusing largely on psychomotor skills and tasks. Levett-Jones et al. (2010, p.64) have also expressed this concern, stating that 'often clinical assessments are focused on psychomotor skills and fail to take into account the multi-dimensional nature of competence and the range of attributes required for clinical practice'. This may relate to a number of factors such as the emphasis placed upon practical skills by the demands of the essential skills clusters (Nursing and Midwifery Council 2007a) and concerns regarding fitness for practice (United Kingdom Central Council

1999). Neither is it surprising that nursing students focus on practical tasks as they want to master the skills that are easily observed. We believe that reflection on carrying out clinical skills can help students to reconnect with the humanistic and wider components of their professional practice.

Harrison and Fopma-Loy go on to propose that nursing education often misses the opportunity to explore how emotions influence decision making and that self-awareness is an undervalued component of reflection. We try to avert this in our own nursing courses where the awareness of emotions is actively promoted and valued because we believe that nurses need to know themselves in order to develop effective relationships and deliver holistic care. It is absolutely necessary to provide the student with a framework that enables them to examine the impact of themselves and their actions upon the whole person. Therefore, helping students to begin to understand the importance of self-awareness and to offer strategies to assist in its development remains an important role of the academic team.

We have acknowledged in previous editions of this chapter that it would be wrong to expect student nurses to become self-aware merely by presenting them with the theory. A good place to start is by asking students to carry out a self-assessment that relates to a particular skill or action. The Practice Assessment Document (PAD) (which is used to record their placement achievements) aims to facilitate this by asking students to take their experiences from taught skills sessions into practice, using the simulated practice learning record sheets, which are discussed in more detail below. Students utilise this as part of the action planning/goal setting with mentors. They should integrate this with the overall goals for achieving their competencies and reflect on the development of that skill as well as the progression towards achieving their clinical competency.

This self-assessment therefore requires self-awareness which is regarded as a life-long skill. To facilitate this, we ask students to carry out written self-assessments in the simulated environment, prior to clinical practice and then in clinical practice. Binding *et al.* (2010) reported that students value the opportunity to integrate reflective writing within simulated activities. This is consistent with our own observation of students at all stages of the nursing programme and supports the view that they should self-assess their clinical practice and competence throughout their course of study (Price 2005; Levett-Jones 2007).

Carrying out a self-assessment will provide the mentor with an indication of the students' self-awareness, which should be fed back to them. Engaging in this dialogue is an expectation of both the mentor and the student and will contribute to the student's evidence for the self-awareness and professional development competencies. Thus, the self-assessment will form part of the student's portfolio of evidence or what the Nursing and Midwifery Council (2008a) refers to as the 'student passport'.

Clinical skills teaching in the 'simulated clinical environment' is becoming increasingly common (e.g. Wilson *et al.* 2005; Ricketts 2010). At Oxford

Chapter 5

Box 5.2   Clinical skills: self-assessment form

Before the activity

- What knowledge do I have of the topic area?
- Where has the knowledge come from?
- What practical experience do I have of this topic area?
- Was I aware of the theory and relevant standards when I practised this in the past?
- What are my hopes in completing these workstations?

After the activity

- What new knowledge have I gained?
- Did I work well with my group and support and share with them?
- How well did I practise my skills?
- What could I have done better?
- What is my plan of action for my future practice with regard to this topic?

Brookes University, the teaching of clinical skills has always been fundamental to practice-related modules and following the Simulation and Practice Learning Project (Nursing and Midwifery Council 2007b); simulated learning activities have been fully incorporated into the curriculum. This work has been led at Oxford Brookes University by Barry Ricketts who published a review of the literature pertaining to simulated learning in the clinical skills laboratory in 2010. For each clinical skills session, students are issued with a simulation and practice learning (SPL) feedback sheet to promote reflection (see Box 5.2).

The questions in the SPL sheet act as triggers that enable the student to identify knowledge, thoughts and assumptions that may guide future learning and critical reflection. It is then used in practice to enable students to communicate what they have learnt to their mentor, to establish SMART (Specific, Measurable, Attainable, Realistic and Timely) goals and objectives in practice, and to provide focus for further reflection. Despite being a good starting point, self-assessment alone does not guarantee self-awareness; therefore students are reminded of the value of checking whether their self-assessment matches the views that others hold and of asking for specific feedback. This process intends to contribute to the process of reflection as described by Gibbs (1988).

It is evident that simulated learning can offer students the opportunity to try out various clinical activities in a safe environment and that this then leads to increased confidence. However, Ricketts (2010) noted that not all students benefit from the same types of learning strategies. What it does suggest is that an opportunity to reflect upon the experience in the skills laboratory and after the session will assist students to gain the most from it, thus supporting Kolb's (1984) concept of experiential learning.

Despite the evident benefits of simulated practice to learners, concerns may remain that students lack the opportunity to experience, understand and prepare for the emotional component of nursing practice. For instance, students may lack the insight to understand the emotional impact of illness upon the patient (Harrison and Fopma-Loy 2010). Acknowledging this potential omission, we integrate reflective activities into the clinical skills teaching so that a more holistic approach is taken in the learning of clinical skills.

In order to further help students develop their self-awareness, we utilise various exercises and activities. Some of the activities are based upon the work of Rungapadiachy (1999) who suggested that there are three dimensions to self-awareness: cognitive (know yourself), behavioural (be yourself) and affective (feel yourself). These dimensions are not independent and will inevitably influence each other. Having an awareness of these concepts will help students to acknowledge and understand how their beliefs, feelings and actions might influence their response to an experience or situation.

During the times when academic advisors meet their students in groups, we draw upon Rungapadiachy's (1999, p.18) dimensions and ask students to identify a situation and consider whether or not their:

- **behaviour** has influenced their **thoughts**
- **thoughts** have influenced their **behaviour**
- **behaviour** has influenced their **feelings**.

In order to enhance students' self-awareness of their clinical skills, audio-visual recording is used to help them to review and reflect upon their practice. For instance, when practising hand-washing techniques, the students are filmed (with their consent). Following the activity, they are asked to reflect on and self-assess their performance. Often they are unaware if they have omitted a stage of the hand-washing procedure. The footage is then played back to the student, which challenges their perception and helps them to realise areas that require more practice as well as what they are doing correctly As a result this activity brings to the surface areas for development.

A pilot study carried out by Grant et al. (2010), which evaluated the impact of using video-facilitated feedback on student performance, demonstrated that it has the potential to improve practice performance. Although not a formal part of the study, Grant et al. report that students valued being able to see their performance on video. This is consistent with our observation of students undertaking the medicines management module at Oxford Brookes University. The students are assessed by an Objective Structured Clinical Examination (OSCE). Those students who need to re-sit the OSCE are shown footage of their exam. Anecdotal feedback suggests that this, along with formal written feedback, is very useful to students. Not only does it enable them to see the areas that require development but it also offers an important insight into their strengths, hence it assists in the development of self-awareness.

Sully and Dallas (2005) say that self-awareness in communication can help us to develop empathy, recognise our perceptions of our clients and cope with distractions, enabling us to develop further the attentive listening skills we need. In both practice and the classroom, students are therefore encouraged to self-assess before any feedback is given in this area. We often need the perspective of another to challenge our self-awareness and Brookfield (2001) has discussed the need to consider different perspectives when exploring our own beliefs and assumptions. However, it is often difficult to step outside our own point of view and the mentor in practice or the classroom facilitator can act as a mirror to the student (Brookfield 2001).

Developing descriptive skills

Helping students to develop their description verbally and in writing is facilitated by asking students to carry out reflection face to face, within the practice assessment document and through formal reflective essays. Several authors advocate the use of diaries, journals and blogs to formally document one's reflection (Jasper 2008; Harrison and Fopma-Loy 2010). However, Harris (2007) acknowledged the difficulties that students may face and suggested that structured support is necessary. It can take time for students to benefit from their writing and there is a risk that they will opt out of reflection if it becomes seen as a largely academic activity. Therefore, helping a student to describe well (verbally and in writing), emphasising that it can improve their professional practice, may help to avoid this.

Whatever means of reflection is used, we find that students tend to focus on feelings within the descriptive stage and often fail to go beyond this. Therefore students need assistance in understanding how to explore the various stages of reflection. Aveyard et al. (2011) suggest that description should involve the presentation of factual information. This is often very difficult when describing a particularly emotive situation. Therefore rather than advising students to remove their feelings from that stage, it is better to advise them on how to present their experience concisely and with clarity (see Chapter 7 for a different view on this). The idea of describing as well as identifying the important issues may be a challenge for some. In many cases, students will describe an event and then move straight on to the conclusion. On raising this, we find that students struggle to understand and utilise the reflective frameworks available to them. As a result, we suggest that they try out the framework described by Driscoll (2007), which offers the basic questions 'What? So what? Now what?'. This framework appears to suit some students because it moves them past the description by asking them what is significant about that experience (So what?) and what are the consequences of exploring that experience (Now what?).

In situations where a student's description is superficial, the teacher or mentor can help them to develop these skills by providing a balance of challenge and support (Daloz 1986). Challenging the student's ideas and assumptions about a situation can help them to identify deeper meaning. Support is also important here to ensure that the student does not feel anxious about what they are being asked to describe, which could result in them withdrawing from the activity. A verbal narrative can be developed in practice, and in the classroom, through the mentor or teacher asking the student to describe events or incidents. The student can be encouraged by a facilitator asking them to 'tell me about it' or 'tell me more about it'. This can help develop students' verbal description skills. This challenge and development of verbal description can then help the student identify what to write in their reflection on practice. In written reflective accounts, the submission of formative work, as discussed in the next section 'the mentor's journey', can help move a learner from description to more analytical and evaluative stages of reflection.

Developing critical analysis and evaluation

Critical analysis invokes fear in many students and is considered hard to grasp. This may be because the word 'critical' suggests that the intention is to find fault or to disapprove. However, analysis of a practice experience should be promoted as a positive activity that involves the breaking down of the event into manageable components in order that it can be more easily examined. Aveyard *et al.* (2011, p.77) have stated that 'analysis can help you to answer questions such as: "What is going on here?", "Why is this happening?" and "What is this about?"'. Cottrell (2005) noted that good critical thinkers often have well-developed self-awareness and so developing this early is crucial to the acquisition of critical analytical skills. Techniques for critical analysis need to be developed as part of a broader range of academic skills and Cottrell (2005) and more recently Aveyard *et al.* (2011) have offered some useful and practical ways in which students can develop this way of thinking, so that they may apply it to their writing. When critically analysing practice, a judgement on the specific event will be made. Often we ask students what was good and bad about the experience. This helps students to start to evaluate in order to identify the most important aspect of that experience. It also helps the student to consider what it is about a situation that might be bothering them, thus providing a focus for subsequent critical analysis.

Gibbs (1988) expands on analysis in his reflective cycle, adding the question: 'What sense can you make of the situation?'. In Chapter 2 of this book Atkins and Schutz suggest that critical analysis should involve identifying existing knowledge, exploration of feelings, challenging of assumptions and the exploration of alternative approaches. Students are helped to develop this skill through academic writing activities, which are then marked using specific grading criteria outlining the requirements. Detailed and focused feedback is essential in order that students may develop these skills as they progress academically. For more discussion about assessing reflection, read Chapter 8 in this book on assessment and evaluation.

It is often helpful for a student to talk through an event, as in critical incident analysis (McGrath and Higgins 2006) or debriefing. The teacher or mentor can adopt the use of 'Socratic questioning' (Elder and Paul 1998) which is an approach designed to uncover the key elements of a problem through systematic questioning. When a teacher adopts this principle of questioning, they aim to check out a student's viewpoint or thinking about a given subject. In this way, such an approach can help to uncover beliefs and assumptions. It can also enable the teacher to check the student's knowledge of a subject and develop critical thinking with the student.

McLoughlin and Darvill (2007) outlined the use of reflection in problem-based learning (PBL), which is an increasingly popular approach to student learning. Within PBL students reflect on the knowledge gained, problem resolution and the effectiveness of working within a group. PBL aims to help students to reflect upon the process of learning as well as the outcome. It is interesting to note that Barrows (1986) referred to the messy practice situations used in PBL and how for healthcare practitioners this connects with real-life situations. This clearly links with Schön's (1983) initial observations about the swampy lowlands of practice problems. Williams (2001) concluded from a review of the literature that practitioners exposed to PBL develop the ability to be reflective in their learning and this skill is developed through a facilitative approach. McLoughlin and Darvill (2007) have also outlined how PBL places practice at the centre of knowledge and learning and how reflection is a strong part of the process. It is clear that PBL uses critical analysis and evaluation and those adopting this approach may further develop these skills.

As we have outlined, the student's journey into reflection is incremental and is facilitated both within the university and within practice settings. We will now discuss how the mentor plays a crucial role in role modelling and facilitating reflection.

The mentor's journey into reflection

Roles and responsibilities

In the wider international literature, the titles and roles of those who support learners in practice have commonalities and differences. In the UK, for nurses and midwives a mentor is defined as an individual who 'facilitates learning, and supervises and assesses students in a practice setting' (Nursing and Midwifery Council 2008a, p.45). In other professions and countries, the title and roles may incorporate some or all of these aspects, such as practice educator, supervisor, clinical educator, preceptor and assessor.

The mentor role includes a wide range of activities (Nursing and Midwifery Council 2008a, p.19) including:

- organising and co-ordinating student learning activities in practice
- supervising students in learning situations and providing them with constructive feedback on their achievements
- setting and monitoring achievement of realistic learning objectives
- assessing total performance including skills, attitudes and behaviours
- providing evidence as required by programme providers of student achievement or lack of achievement
- liaising with others to provide feedback, identify any concerns about the students' performance and agree action as appropriate
- providing evidence for, or acting as sign-off mentors with regard to making decisions about achievement of proficiency at the end of a programme.

All this outlines what is a complex and challenging role for staff whose key responsibility is for patient/client care.

In order to help mentors to understand their responsibilities, the Nursing and Midwifery Council (2008a, pp.20–21) has identified a developmental framework as part of its *Standards to Support Learning and Assessment in Practice*, moving from registrant (nurses and midwives) to mentor, practice teacher and then teacher. It details this for each of these roles in eight domains.

1. Establishing effective working relationships
2. Facilitation of learning
3. Assessment and accountability
4. Evaluation of learning
5. Creating an environment for learning
6. Context of practice
7. Evidence-based practice
8. Leadership.

The standards have been in place since 2006 with an updated version in 2008 with several circulars to clarify some complex interpretations. The only mention of reflection in the actual domains is under the heading 'Facilitation of learning' where it is stated that mentors need to: 'Support students in *critically reflecting* upon their learning experiences in order to enhance future learning' (Nursing and Midwifery Council 2008a, p.20).

It is disappointing that the value of reflection is not developed in other domains and although it is a very broad statement, the significance of it should not be lost. Indeed, it acknowledges that mentors do have a role in supporting students in their critical reflections and this could be in a variety of ways which we will discuss. It also alludes to the notion that reflection will impact on learning.

Chapter 5

Box 5.3   Record of meetings between sign-off mentor and student at Oxford Brookes University (OBU) Practice Assessment Document (PAD) (OBU 2012)

Sign-off mentor feedback and declaration to be completed at the end of the last 12 weeks of professional practice

Year of study:	Semester:	Placement:
Sign-off mentor name:		Link lecturer name:

Record of sign-off mentor's protected time (this is for feedback and reflective activities, regular discussions and review of progress. This should be at least 1 hour per 37.5 hours of student practice equivalence)

There is the additional role of sign-off mentor (SOM) which applies to those who meet additional criteria and who will validate the final competence in nursing students who are about to qualify. The standards do state that the SOM should have *time to reflect*, give feedback and keep records. In our organisation, we have developed a system to record these meetings (see Box 5.3). There is an allocated 1 hour per week for this activity. As finding sufficient time for reflection has been identified by practitioners as problematic (Mamede and Schmidt 2005), this could be monitored by those in leadership positions at significant points of the placement, such as mid-way meetings.

In addition to the standards produced by the Nursing and Midwifery Council, the Royal College of Nursing (2007, p.5) has produced guidance for mentors of student nurses and midwives and reports that 'the role of the mentor is to *facilitate reflection* on practice, performance and experiences' and that mentors are responsible for providing time for this reflection and feedback. It also recognises that mentors should *reflect on the role* themselves in order to develop.

The role of reflection in mentor development

As professionals, practitioners should continue their development from the moment they qualify. Those who have developed confidence and skill in using reflection are likely to find this helpful once they qualify. We discussed at the start of this chapter the importance of reflection as a key component of clinical judgement, decision making, accountability and critical thinking that can help practitioners in their professional practice.

It is our view that thinking and reflective nurses are likely to become thinking and reflective mentors.

As well as reflecting for the benefit of their professional growth, clinical practice and development, mentors may need to provide evidence of their own development as mentors and reflective activities can help with this. In the UK mentors should update annually (Nursing and Midwifery Council 2008a). There are various ways in which mentors can generate this evidence and some of these areas overlap with approaches used by students and are discussed further below.

Mentor preparation and reflection

At about a year after qualifying, nurses and midwives are encouraged to prepare to become a mentor. In the UK, 10 days are allocated for completion of mentor preparation programmes; five of these are protected learning time and five can be work-based learning. It is challenging in the current pressured environment for prospective mentors to given the allocated time or supervision. The Nursing and Midwifery Council (2008a) mentions that mentor preparation programmes should include opportunities for prospective mentors to practise mentoring activities under the supervision of a qualified mentor and 'have the opportunity to *critically reflect* on such an experience' (p.29). It does not, however, define what it means by critical reflection.

Brookfield (2009) discusses the concept of critical reflection and identifies that it is distinct from reflection *per se* as it moves from focusing on process to challenging and uncovering assumptions. In earlier work, Brookfield (1988) identified activities that are central to critical reflection.

- Assumption analysis – this involves challenging beliefs, values, cultural practices and social structures so that we can evaluate their impact.
- Contextual awareness – this involves recognition that our assumptions are based within historical, social, personal and cultural contexts.
- Imaginative speculation – this involves thinking in alternative ways to our usual approaches.
- Reflective scepticism – this encompasses temporarily rejecting or disbelieving current evidence in order to think about the feasibility of other suggestions or approaches.

Having an experienced mentor/practice teacher to help the developing mentor to undertake critical reflection as part of their ongoing development would undoubtedly be valuable. We have developed a tool with reflective trigger questions to facilitate critical reflection. It is structured around the detail of the Nursing and Midwifery Council's (2008a) eight domains at stage 2 (for mentors). These detailed reflective triggers can also be used to help with self-assessment which is needed as part of a

Chapter 5

triennial review of the mentor's role (Nursing and Midwifery Council 2008a) or as a stimulus for reflective discussions with an experienced mentor as part of the work-based learning part of mentor development.

Reflective trigger questions based on the Nursing and Midwifery Council eight domains

Under Domain 1: Establishing effective relationships

- How well do I understand what impacts on the student's integration into the placement setting?
- How well do I support the student and recognise the differences between students and placement settings?
- What influences the success of relationships with students for me? Do I have any preconceived ideas, what are my beliefs and values in relation to what is a 'good student'? Have I considered wider issues such as culture, age, gender, power, etc.?
- Have I fully considered how the relationships with myself and other members of the team might impact on student learning and assessment?

For all of the above: How do I know? How do I feel? How can I improve?

Under Domain 2: Creating an environment for learning

- How well do I help students to set goals that are relevant to their level and experiences, and what influences my own expectations?
- How creative am I in identifying a range of opportunities for students, including colleagues and clients, and do any of my own preferences or lack of interest influence what I select?
- How well do I recognise the factors that influence the learning environment on the individual student experience?
- How fully do I act as a resource to students and colleagues? How do I react and behave when I don't know something?

For all of the above: How do I know? How do I feel? How can I improve?

Under Domain 3: Facilitation of learning, evidence-based practice and context for practice

- How well do I select learning experiences based on the level the student is at and their personal interests? What do I favour and what do I avoid? What influences my choices?
- Do I use a full range of approaches to facilitate student learning, integrating theory and practice?
- How well do I help students to reflect on their learning experiences in a critical way? Do I successfully use any frameworks to enhance this process?

For all of the above: How do I know? How do I feel? How can I improve?

Under Domain 4: Evidence-based practice

- Where do I access information for my practice from?
- How well do I access and use research and evidence-based practice in my area of practice? Are my skills up to date in searching, appraising and implementing evidence?
- How can I work with colleagues to increase or review the evidence base used to support practice?
- What is my awareness of the relevance of any National Service Frameworks, NICE guidelines, policy and guidelines used in my sphere of practice? What are my beliefs about knowledge for practice and how does this influence my role with students?
- What is my attitude to learning from students and how can I better support them in using best available evidence?

For all of the above: How do I know? How do I feel? How can I improve?

Under Domain 5: Context for practice

- How do I ensure that the student is witnessing, and role modelling from, effective practice within the placement area? What factors may currently be influencing the learning environment (e.g. change, morale, conflicts)?
- In my own and others' professional roles, are relationships clear to the student? Do the professional and interprofessional relationships/ dynamics/boundaries contribute to the success of care delivery? What is the student's perspective?
- Do I implement and respond to practice developments to ensure safe and effective care is achieved? How do I react to challenges to the way I do things and how do I respond to potential and actual change? Do I invite challenge and questioning of my practice?

For all of the above: How do I know? How do I feel? How can I improve?

Under Domain 6: Assessment and accountability

- How well do I help students to develop personally and professionally, taking on appropriate responsibility and accountability?
- How up to date am I regarding assessment approaches? Is my assessment of the student fair, transparent, rigorous and consistent? What is my attitude to assessment and does my relationship with the student have any influence?
- How effective am I at providing constructive feedback and goal/objective setting in relation to student performance and development?

- What do I feel about managing an underperforming student? How effectively might I manage a failing student? Do I seek support appropriately?
- Do I recognise my own accountability for confirming that students have met, or not met, the Nursing and Midwifery Council competencies in practice and as a sign-off mentor? How do I see my role in relation to safeguarding the profession?

For all of the above: How do I know? How do I feel? How can I improve?

Under Domain 7: Evaluation of learning

- How do I evaluate the experience of the student learning and assessment experiences? Do I invite feedback?
- How well do I self-assess and invite personal and professional feedback on my performance in the role of mentor and as a professional?
- What is my attitude to evaluating the performance of others? Do I professionally and constructively challenge poor practice and praise good practice?

For all of the above: How do I know? How do I feel? How can I improve?

Under Domain 8: Leadership

- How well do I plan the students' learning experiences to meet their needs?
- Do I act on behalf of students, helping them to access a wide range of learning opportunities and to contact other professionals, patients, clients and carers? What influences my choices?
- How well do I manage/prioritise my own workload to enable me to effectively support students?
- How might I constructively feed back to the university and to my managers about the effectiveness of learning and assessment in practice? Am I aware of and do I contribute to formal evaluation processes?

For all of the above: How do I know? How do I feel? How can I improve?

Additional reflective approaches that can be used by mentors

Mentors are able to use reflection for their own development as well as an approach for facilitating and assessing student learning. When they show students that they personally reflect, they are modelling that they are thinking and learning from their own practice experiences. A key part of learning in practice comes from role modelling (Cruess *et al.* 2008; Perry 2009), and reflection on what has been observed is a crucial part of this process.

Cruess *et al.* (2008) offer strategies to improve role modelling and the mentor's role in facilitating reflection is part of this.

- Be aware of being a role model
- Be clinically competent
- Protect time for teaching
- Be positive in your attitude
- Be student centred
- Facilitate reflection on clinical experiences and what has been modelled
- Talk to colleagues
- Be involved in staff development
- Develop the culture of the organisation

Verbal approaches to reflection

In busy practice situations, mentors may find it useful to use verbal approaches with colleagues or students. The quickest approach is to reflect on what was good about a patient care episode or issue and what could be improved. Mentors could ask students to do this following any care episode, or prior to undertaking an episode of care where they could reflect on previous experiences. Some of the more concise frameworks such as Gibbs (1988) or Driscoll (2007) may be of use in structuring verbal reflections.

Approaches such as debriefing (Dreifuerst 2009; Arafeh *et al.* 2010) or reflective one-to-one discussions can be useful. Manning *et al.* (2009) described how reflective groups for some students in practice helped support their experience and at times gave them different perspectives. Newton (2011) also discussed the benefits of group reflection in helping student nurses to challenge their assumptions and values and become more prepared for professional practice. Action learning sets (Currie *et al.* 2012) that can be focused on a particular incident or general issue can also be used and in some cases can help professionals deal with challenging or emotional issues (see Chapter 4 for more help on reflecting in groups). Mentors may also suggest to students that they reflect on certain practice issues or elements of a certain competency, before a more structured discussion or feedback takes place. This can be particularly useful if the mentor has concerns about a student's performance in practice.

Some professional groups use clinical supervision as a means of guided reflection for professional growth and development (Johns 2010). Supervision is perhaps more widely used in mental health nursing (Bradshaw *et al.* 2007) and midwifery. Practitioners may prefer to identify a 'critical friend' to help them reflect, defined as 'a trusted person who asks provocative questions, provides data to be examined through another lens, and offers critiques of a person's work ...' (Costa and Kallick 1993). Appleton (2008) adds that a critical friend should be both challenging and supporting and ask key questions to promote deeper analysis.

Although it is worth noting that clinical supervision is not intended to be part of the appraisal process, mentors who have participated in this type of developmental activity are more likely to be able to provide an account of their own development. This fits in well with the Nursing and Midwifery Council (2008a) standards and need for mentors to have a triennial review of their mentoring activities. There is also an increasing uptake of digital forums for reflective discussion, electronic portfolios in practice (Bogossian et al. 2009) and dialogue such as blogs or discussion boards that bridge the gap between verbal and written approaches. It is important that strict care is taken to ensure confidential and professional narratives.

Written approaches to reflection

Reflective accounts can of course be captured in writing such as in reflective journals/diaries, critical incident analyses, reflective self-assessment, reflective learning contracts or in writing reflective essays for more formal assessments (as outlined below). Walsh (2010) discusses how experiential learning, critical incident analysis and portfolios all use reflection. He explains how experiential learning is learning by doing and then reflecting on it – referring back to Kolb's (1984) experiential learning cycle. Walsh also warns about lengthy reflective writing in practice that can easily lose focus. In our own institution we have moved from lengthy reflective learning contracts to more succinct focused reflective accounts in the students' practice assessment documents (PAD).

A reflective essay as part of mentor course assessment

When writing reflectively, there is overlap with general academic writing skills because the elements of description, analysis, evaluation and conclusion are part of writing reflectively. Aveyard et al. (2011, Chapter 4) recognised this overlap and have outlined some of the distinct features of different types of writing. In both pre- and post-qualifying courses a reflective essay may be the assignment of choice as it can link theory and practice and demonstrate personal growth and development. (Exemplars from nursing students' reflective essays can be found in Chapter 9.)

At Oxford Brookes University, the mentor preparation programme has a summative assignment that requires writing a reflective essay entitled: 'Critical reflection on my facilitation of learning: including reflection on the observation, and my learning from the module overall'. The aim of the assignment is to help mentors become familiar with, or develop further, their own reflective skills and in the process demonstrate that they have incorporated some of the key elements of the module into their own practice. We explain the advantages of reflection and provide an example of reflective writing.

Those undertaking the course explore various reflective frameworks and discuss the skills for reflection. However, many of these qualified nurses have either not used reflection at all or not for some time, others have used it as part of their pre-registration programmes but all express anxiety about writing reflectively. Mentors can select a reflective framework of their choice and as facilitators of this course, we constantly verbalise our own reflections on the facilitation process – thereby modelling how reflection on practice can be used. As a facilitator of this course, one of us recalls that:

> 'I have shared personal reflection on my own learning and performance, so role modelling what mentors themselves are being asked to do. The elusive skills of analysis, evaluation and synthesis are also role modelled in the classroom (for example, when referring to educational theory or definitions they will be 'pulled apart', compared and their sources critiqued). I may end a session by reflecting on what I think went well; what I may change for next time'.

The idea behind this is that the participants will see how verbalising learning and reflecting on one's own performance can help others to learn. It is intended that they will see the value of role modelling and do this in their own practice with their learners.

The value of dialogue in reflective writing
The aim of this reflective essay is that those undertaking the course need to think critically about what they have learnt. However, their early writing can be overly descriptive and tends to separate out the theory from their experiences. This is where a formative assessment really helps; the students are allowed to submit 1000 words of their reflective writing for feedback at the mid-way point and the facilitators can then add prompts or ask challenging questions, such as: 'Why do you think that?', 'What influences this perspective?' and they suggest areas where improvements can be made. This formative dialogue between the assessor and the mentor really helps the development of more critical reflection. From this feedback process and our experience of helping mentors develop, we have generated several ideas to help with reflective writing.

- If you describe feelings, say what has influenced the feelings – *for example, if you say you felt nervous about meeting a student for the first time, think what reasons there are for the nervousness and what has influenced them.*
- Consider the feelings of others in the situation – *consider how you know what they felt or what assumptions you might have made and why.*
- Ensure theory is not just described but applied, and where possible appraised. For example, many mentors reflect upon assessing the learning style or preference of the student using tools such as VARK

(Fleming 2001–2011) which categorises learners' preferences for visual, aural, read/write or kinaesthetic styles of learning. However, in their initial writings they may not have fully considered the value of these tools or the evidence behind them and their value can be questioned (Scott 2010). The key message is don't just accept what you read, think about it more deeply to ensure you reflect critically.

- Consider the reflective trigger questions based on the Nursing and Midwifery Council's (2008a) eight domains for mentors, described above.

Examples of how reflective writing has helped mentors' development
Some students will really move from descriptive writing towards deeper learning and gain a clear 'perspective transformation' if they adopt a more critically reflective approach (Platzer *et al.* 2000; Glaze 2001). As an example, one nurse had always mentored learners in the way that she liked to be supported herself. She had never considered the individuality of the student, preferences for learning or the issue of power. She reflected in depth on this topic and had an 'ah ha!' moment when she realised there may be other ways of supporting students that she had not considered before. She began to question her own assumptions and perspectives in depth and became open to new ideas, thus showing the beginnings of more critical reflection and perspective transformation.

Reflecting on their own performance and observing more experienced facilitators has helped many mentors to see how they have previously adopted a very teacher-orientated, rather than student-focused approach to facilitating learning – supplying the answers to students' questions and not embracing the principles of active, adult learning. This became more apparent when mentors saw (through facilitator example) that learning became more interesting when the facilitator challenged the student and got them to find out, do or suggest things. They reflected on how this would change their approach in the future.

Another student wrote her essay about student motivation. She stated that the main learning for her had been from reflection on her own motivation as a student and that this had moved her focus to a wider perspective than that covered in the module. She developed her essay by drawing on her initial reluctance to attend the course, how the enthusiasm and personality of the facilitator put her at ease, and how she found a new interest and knowledge about how she could make the lives of her students more interesting and stimulating. The value of structured reflection here was that she learnt something unexpected from the course, above and beyond the content.

Zannini *et al.* (2011), in a small qualitative study in Italy, described how mentors were assessed following a mentor preparation course. They undertook an assignment entitled 'Writing a letter to yourself'. This reflective letter identified that almost all participants felt 'profoundly changed and experienced a sense of personal and professional growth' (Zannini *et al.* 2011, p.1806). In an article written from the mentor's perspective,

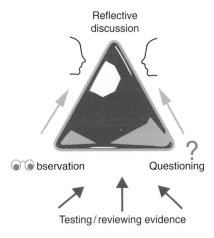

Reflective
discussion

bservation   Questioning

Testing / reviewing evidence

Figure 5.1   Reflection as part of the assessment process. (Based on Driscoll and O'Sullivan 2007, p.6)

McNair *et al.* (2007) described the experience of a mentor using a critical incident as a trigger to explore learning when undertaking a mentor preparation course. They described how the increased knowledge gained from the course, together with reflection on the experience of being mentored, had allowed the mentor to feel much more prepared for the role. All these examples show how for many mentors, the processes involved in reflection have helped them move from surface to deeper learning as has been previously identified by Moon (1999).

Reflection and its place in student assessment

Assessment is one of the key roles of a mentor and can be one that causes most anxiety. Competency statements often contain reference to knowledge, skills and attitudes (National Nursing Research Unit 2009) and reflection can be used in all these areas. It can be useful before or after observation of clinical and professional skills and behaviours, and reflective discussions, questioning, and review of reflective writing can be used to assess knowledge and attitudes (Figure 5.1).

As in any assessment, it is important that there is rigour and fairness. In a discussion paper with a case example, Cassidy (2009) describes 'valid subjectivity' where an assessment is made from a position of trust and commitment. He proposes that humanistic approaches such as reflection and examination of thoughts and feelings can provide opportunities to assess. He discusses (p.36) how 'reflection as action stimulates a continual reframing and re-evaluation of the event, prompting further action and new reflection' and he demonstrates this in a personal account of an encounter between himself and a student.

Within education establishments and practice settings, we should ensure that where reflection is used in assessing practice learning, the purpose and process are fully explained to students and mentors. This is important so that mentors are clear about whether they are assessing the student's reflection alone, or if they are assessing practice using reflection *as a tool*. In our pre-registration course, the students use reflection as a tool and can reflect verbally or in writing in their practice assessment document to provide evidence of competency. However, McCready (2007) highlighted the challenges of using such portfolios as part of the assessment of competence and recommended clear guidelines for their use.

Reflection is part of experiential learning and so as students observe and then practise their clinical skills, mentors can observe them, and their personal reflection on their learning can become part of the evidence for assessment. Duffy's (2003) seminal qualitative research highlighted why mentors continue to find assessment of competency difficult, particularly with poorly performing students. She identified lack of confidence, concern about emotional response and lack of skill or support as some of the reasons. Mentors may find reflecting on their experience of supporting a failing student valuable because they can explore their experiences in more depth and learn from them.

Conclusion

This chapter has identified the value of reflection to both students and mentors in supporting them to face some of the challenges in practice education. We have explored how reflection is a key component of clinical judgement, accountability and critical thinking. We have outlined how reflection equips students with a way of developing self-awareness and integrating theory in either simulated or real practice. The skills for reflective practice are developed over time, and we have suggested that appropriate tools and support for reflection are needed by students. We have also emphasised that reflection should be part of mentors' own development and then role modelled to their students. We have offered verbal and written reflective approaches that mentors can use, including 'trigger questions' based on the Nursing and Midwifery Council (2008a) standards, and suggested key ways in which mentors can further develop their approaches to reflection. In summary, we have illustrated how the development and use of reflection are valuable to both the students' and mentors' personal development and ongoing achievement of thoughtful and excellent professional practice.

References

Appleton, J. (2008) Using reflection in a palliative care educational programme. In: Bulman, C. and Schutz, S. (eds) *Reflective Practice in Nursing*, 4th edn. Wiley-Blackwell, Oxford.

Arafeh, J.M., Hansen S.S. and Nichols, A. (2010) Debriefing in simulated-based learning: Facilitating a reflective discussion. *Journal of Perinatal and Neonatal Nursing*, **24**(4), 302–309.

Atkins, S. and Schutz, S. (2008) Developing the skills for reflective practice. In: Bulman, C. and Schutz, S. (eds) *Reflective Practice in Nursing*, 4th edn. Wiley-Blackwell, Oxford.

Aveyard, H., Sharp, P. and Woolliams, M. (2011) *A Beginner's Guide to Critical Thinking in Health and Social Care*. Open University Press, Buckingham.

Barrows, H. (1986) A taxonomy of problem based learning. *Medical Education*, **20**(6), 481–486.

Binding, L., Morck, A. and Moules, N. (2010) Learning to see the other: a vehicle of reflection. *Nurse Education Today*, **30**(6), 591–594.

Bogossian, F.E., Kellett, S.E.M. and Mason, B. (2009) The use of tablet PCs to access an electronic portfolio in the clinical setting: a pilot study using undergraduate nursing students. *Nurse Education Today*, **29**(2), 246–253.

Bradshaw, T., Butterworth, A. and Mairs, H. (2007) Does structured clinical supervision during psychosocial intervention education enhance outcome for mental health nurses and the service users they work with? *Journal of Psychiatric and Mental Health Nursing*, **14**(1), 4–12.

Brookfield, S. (1988) Developing critically reflective practitioners: a rationale for training educators of adults. In: Brookfield, S. (ed) *Training Educators of Adults: The Theory and Practice of Graduate Adult Education*. Routledge, New York.

Brookfield, S.D. (2001) *Developing Critical Thinkers: Challenging Adults to Explore Alternative Ways of Thinking and Acting*, 5th edn. Open University Press, Buckingham.

Brookfield, S.D. (2009) The concept of critical reflection: promises and contradictions. *European Journal of Social Work*, **12**, 293–304.

Bulman, C. (2008) An introduction to reflection. In: Bulman, C. and Schutz, S. (eds) *Reflective Practice in Nursing*, 4th edn. Wiley-Blackwell, Oxford.

Cassidy, S. (2009) Subjectivity and the valid assessment of pre-registration student nurse clinical learning outcomes: implications for mentors. *Nurse Education Today*, **29**(1), 33–39.

Costa, A.L. and Kallick, B. (1993) Through the lens of a critical friend. *Educational Leadership*, **51**(2), 49–51.

Cottrell, S. (2005) *Critical Thinking Skills: Developing Effective Analysis and Argument*. Palgrave Macmillan, New York.

Cruess, S.R., Cruess, R.L. and Steinert, Y. (2008) Role modeling – making the most of a powerful teaching tool. *British Medical Journal*, **336**(7646), 718–721.

Currie, K., Biggam, J., Palmer, J. and Corcoran, T. (2012) Participants' engagement with and reactions to the use of on-line action learning sets to support advanced nursing role development. *Nurse Education Today*, **32**(3), 267–272.

Daloz, L. (1986) *Effective Teaching and Mentoring: Realizing the Transformational Power of Adult Learning Experiences*. Jossey-Bass, San Francisco.

Dreifuerst, K.T. (2009) The essentials of debriefing in simulation learning: a concept analysis. *Nursing Education Perspectives*, **30**(2), 109–114.

Driscoll, J. (2007) *Practising Clinical Supervision: A Reflective Approach for Healthcare Professionals*. Baillière Tindall, Elsevier, Edinburgh.

Chapter 5

Duffy, K. (2003) Failing Students. www.nmcuk.org/documents/Archived%20 Publications/1Research%20papers/Kathleen_Duffy_Failing_Students2003.pdf

Eckroth-Bucher, M. (2010) Self-awareness: a review and analysis of a basic nursing concept. *Advances in Nursing Science*, **33**(4), 297–309.

Elder, L. and Paul, R. (1998) The role of Socratic questioning in thinking, teaching and learning. *The Clearing House*, **71**(5), 297–301.

Facione, P.A. (2011) *Think Critically.* Pearson Education, Englewood Cliffs, NJ.

Fleming, N. (2001–2011) VARK: A guide to learning styles. www.vark-learn.com

Fowler, J. (2008) Experiential learning and its facilitation. *Nurse Education Today*, **28**(4), 427–433.

Gibbs, G., Farmer, B. and Eastcott, D. (1988) *Learning by Doing. A Guide to Teaching and Learning Methods.* Far Eastern University, Birmingham Polytechnic.

Glaze, J.E. (2001) Reflection as a transforming process: student advanced nurse practitioners' experiences of developing reflective skills as part of an MSc programme. *Journal of Advanced Nursing*, **34**(5), 639–647.

Gopee, N. (2011) *Mentoring and Supervision in Healthcare*, 2nd edn. Sage Publications Ltd, London.

Grant, J., Moss, J., Epps, C. and Watts, P. (2010) Using video-facilitated feedback to improve student performance following high-fidelity simulation. *Clinical Simulation in Nursing*, **6**, 177–184.

Harris, M. (2007) Scaffolding reflective journal writing – negotiating power, play and position. *Nurse Education Today*, **28**(3), 314–326.

Harrison, P.A. and Fopma-Loy, J.L. (2010) Reflective journal prompts: a vehicle for stimulating emotional competence in nursing. *Journal of Nursing Education*, **49**(11), 644–652.

Higgs, J. and Jones, M.A. (2000) *Clinical Reasoning in the Health Professions*, 2nd edn. Butterworth-Heinemann, Oxford.

Jasper, M. (2006) *Professional Development, Reflection and Decision Making.* Wiley-Blackwell, Oxford.

Jasper, M. (2008) Using reflective journals and diaries to enhance practice and learning. In: Bulman, C. and Schutz, S. (eds) *Reflective Practice in Nursing*, 4th edn. Wiley-Blackwell, Oxford.

Johns, C. (2010) Clinical supervision: reflective practice; learning through experience. In: Cox, C. and Hill, M. (eds) *Professional Issues in Primary Care Nursing.* Wiley-Blackwell, Oxford.

Kolb, D.A. (1984) *Experiential Learning. Experience as a Source of Learning and Development.* Prentice-Hall, New Jersey.

Levett-Jones, T.L. (2007) Facilitating reflective practice and self-assessment of competence through the use of narratives. *Nurse Education in Practice*, **7**(2), 112–119.

Levett-Jones, T.L., Gerbasch, J., Arthur, C. and Roche, J. (2010) Implementing a clinical competency assessment model that promotes critical reflection and ensures nursing graduates' readiness for professional practice. *Nurse Education in Practice*, **11**(1), 64–69.

Magnusson, C., O'Driscoll, M. and Smith, P. (2007) New roles to support practice learning – can they facilitate expansion of placement capacity? *Nurse Education Today*, **27**(6), 643–650.

Mallik, M. and McGowan, B. (2007) Issues in practice based learning in nursing in the United Kingdom and the Republic of Ireland: results from a multi-professional scoping exercise. *Nurse Education Today*, **27**(1), 52–59.

Mamede, S. and Schmidt, H. (2005) Correlates of reflective practice in medicine. *Advances in Health Sciences Education, Theory and Practice*, **10**(4), 327–337.

Mann, K., Gordon, J. and MacLeod, A. (2009) Reflection and reflective practice in health professions education: a systematic review. *Advances in Health Science Education*, **14**(4), 595–621.

Manning, A., Cronin, P., Monaghan, A. and Rawlings-Anderson, K. (2009) Supporting students in practice: an exploration of reflective groups as a means of support. *Nurse Education in Practice*, **9**(3), 176–183.

Mantzoukas, S. and Jasper, M. (2008) Types of nursing knowledge used to guide care of hospitalized patients. *Journal of Advanced Nursing*, **62**(3), 318–326.

Matthew, C. and Sternberg, R. (2009) Developing experience-based (tacit) knowledge through reflection. *Learning and Individual Differences*, **19**(4), 530–540.

McCready, T. (2007) Portfolios and the assessment of competence in nursing: a literature review. *International Journal of Nursing Studies*, **44**(1), 143–151.

McGrath, D. and Higgins, A. (2006) Implementing and evaluating reflective practice group sessions. *Nurse Education in Practice*, **6**(3), 175–181.

McLoughlin, M. and Darvill, A. (2007) Peeling back the layers of learning: a classroom model for problem-based learning. *Nurse Education Today*, **27**(4), 271–277.

McNair, W., Smith, B. and Ellis, J. (2007) A vision of mentorship in practice. *Journal of Perioperative Practice*, **17**(9), 421–430.

Moon, J. (1999) *Reflection in Learning and Professional Development*. Kogan Page, London.

Morris, J. and Stew, G. (2007) Collaborative reflection: how far do 2:1 models of learning in the practice setting promote peer reflection? *Reflective Practice: International and Multidisciplinary Perspectives*, **8**(3), 419–432.

National Nursing Research Unit (2009) Nursing competence: what are we assessing and how should it be measured? *Policy Plus* no.118. www.kcl.ac.uk/content/1/c6/05/68/69/PolicyIssue18.pdf

Newton, J.M. (2011) Reflective learning groups for nursing students. *Professional and Practice-based Learning*, **7**(1), 119–130.

Nursing and Midwifery Council (2007a) *Introduction of Essential Skills Clusters for Pre-Registration Nursing Programmes*. Circular 07/07 plus annexe 1 and annexe 2. Nursing and Midwifery Council, London. www.nmcuk.org/Documents/Circulars/2007circulars/NMCcircular07_2007.pdf

Nursing and Midwifery Council (2007b) *Supporting Direct Care through Simulated Practice Learning in the Pre-registration Nursing Programme*. Nursing and Midwifery Council, London. www.nmcuk.org/Documents/Circulars/2007circulars/NMCcircular36_2007.pdf

Nursing and Midwifery Council (2008a) *Standard to Support Learning and Assessment in Practice*. Nursing and Midwifery Council, London. www.nmcuk.org/Publications/Standards/

Nursing and Midwifery Council (2008b) *The Code: Standards of Conduct, Performance and Ethics for Nurses and Midwives*. Nursing and Midwifery Council, London. www.nmcuk.org/Publications/Standards/

Chapter 5

Nursing and Midwifery Council (2009) *Accountability*. Nursing and Midwifery Council, London. www.nmcuk.org/Nurses-and-midwives/Advice-by-topic/A/Advice/Accountability/

O'Donovan, M. (2006) Reflecting during clinical placement – discovering factors that influence pre-registration psychiatric nursing students. *Nurse Education in Practice*, **6**(3), 134–140.

O'Regan, H. and Fawcett, T. (2006) Learning to nurse: reflections on bathing a patient. *Nursing Standard*, **20**(46), 60–64.

Parker, I. (1997) *Psychoanalytic Culture: Psychoanalytic Discourse in Western Society*. Sage Publications, London.

Perry, B. (2009) Role modelling excellence in clinical nursing practice. *Nurse Education in Practice*, **9**(1), 36–44.

Platzer, H., Blake, D. and Ashford, D. (2000) An evaluation of the process and outcome of learning through reflective practice groups on a post-registration nursing course. *Journal of Advanced Nursing*, **31**(3), 689–695.

Price, B. (2005) Thinking aloud your practice: mentoring learners in practice. *Nursing Standard*, Supplement 8, **19**(31), 73–74.

Ricketts, B. (2011) The role of simulation for learning within pre-registration nursing education – a literature review. *Nurse Education Today*, **31**(7), 650–654.

Royal College of Nursing (2006) *Helping Students Get the Best From Their Practice Placements*. Royal College of Nursing, London. www.rcn.org.uk/__data/assets/pdf_file/0011/78545/001815.pdf

Royal College of Nursing (2007) *Guidance for Mentors of Nursing Students and Midwives*, 2nd edn. Royal College of Nursing, London. www.rcn.org.uk/__data/assets/pdf_file/0008/78677/002797.pdf

Royal College of Nursing (2011) *Nurses Struggle as Staffing Pressures Bite, says Royal College of Nursing*. Royal College of Nursing, London. www.rcn.org.uk/newsevents/press_releases/uk/nurses_struggle_as_staffing_pressures_bite,_says_royal_college_of_nursing

Rungapadiachy, D. (1999) *Interpersonal Communication and Psychology for Healthcare Professionals*. Butterworth-Heinemann, Oxford.

Schön, D. (1983) *The Reflective Practitioner: How Professionals Think in Action*. Basic Books, London.

Schön, D. (1987) *Educating the Reflective Practitioner: Towards a New Design for Teaching and Learning in the Professions*. Jossey-Bass, San Francisco.

Scott, C. (2010) The enduring appeal of learning styles. *Australian Journal of Education*, **54**(1), 5–17.

Somerville, D. and Keeling, J. (2004) A practical approach to promote reflective practice within nursing. *Nursing Times*, **100**(12), 42–45.

Sully, P. and Dallas, J. (2005) *Essential Communication Skills for Nursing Practice*. Elsevier Mosby, Philadelphia.

Teekman, B. (2000) Exploring reflective thinking in nursing practice. *Journal of Advanced Nursing*, **31**(5), 1125–1135.

Triggle, N. and Hughes, J. (2011) Nearly 50,000 jobs 'under threat'. www.bbc.co.uk/news/health-15780965

United Kingdom Central Council (1999) *Fitness for Practice*. United Kingdom Central Council, London.

Walsh, D. (2010) *The Nurse Mentor's Handbook: Supporting Students in Clinical Practice*. Open University Press, Buckingham.

Williams, B. (2001) Developing critical reflection for professional practice through problem-based learning. *Journal of Advanced Nursing*, **34**(1), 27–34.

Wilson, A. (2010) Are the demands of nurse mentoring underestimated? www.nursingtimes.net/are-the-demands-of-nurse-mentoring-underestimated/5015817.article

Wilson, M., Shepherd, I., Kelly, C. and Pitzner, J. (2005) Assessment of low fidelity human patient simulator for the acquisition of nursing skills. *Nurse Education Today*, **25**(1), 56–67.

Zannini, L., Cattaneo, C., Brugnolli, A. and Saiani, L. (2011) How do healthcare professionals perceive themselves after a mentoring programme? A qualitative study based on the reflective exercise of 'writing a letter to yourself'. *Journal of Advanced Nursing*, **67**(8), 1800–1810.

Chapter 5

Chapter 6

Supervision for supervisors: icing on the cake or a basic ingredient for the development of clinical supervision in nursing?

John Driscoll[1] and Paul Cassedy[2]
[1]Freelance CPD Consultant and Coach, Norfolk, UK
[2]School of Nursing, University of Nottingham, Nottingham, UK

Introduction

The title of this chapter at first glance may not seem that controversial. The cake metaphor refers to the ingredients required for the often complex implementation of nursing clinical supervision (CS) in healthcare organisations. The development of those engaged in the CS relationship, and in particular the clinical supervisory role, is a key part of that recipe and, it would seem, critical for the initiative to be sustained in clinical practice. Perhaps you as the reader and a working clinical supervisor (or supervisee) will readily agree with this as part of the process following your implementation of CS. However, we wonder how many active clinical supervisors in the milieu of busy practice as clinicians take time out to reflect on *supervisory practice*. What may be more likely is that valuable CS time as a practitioner involves reflecting on significant issues directly related to the rigours and tensions of delivering clinical practice, rather than being a working clinical supervisor. Against this backdrop, both John and Paul (as authors), who have many years of experience in implementing CS as well as facilitating clinical supervisor programmes, decided to investigate what sorts of things might be discussed in CS as supervisors.

The plethora of available literature and debate about what and how CS is utilised in nursing practice contrasts sharply with the lack of debate regarding the supervision of supervisors and the implications of this for the longer term development of CS in nursing practice. Whilst Arvidsson and Fridlund (2005) consider the supervision of supervisors as essential, Williams and Irvine's (2009) study suggests that working supervisors also valued other methods of support such as mentoring and working within a supervisor peer group. Milne (2009, p.154) also laments that whilst in professional circles the emphasis on engaging in CS is resounding, how supervisors might be supported to carry out their work in healthcare remains muted. He was referring to his own discipline of clinical psychology, but the same may apply in nursing. Indeed, Sloan (2006, p.138) in an extensive CS study in mental health nursing noted how after some introductory training, clinical supervisors in many settings throughout the UK were then left to get on with the task of delivering CS with limited opportunities for support and further development.

This chapter aims to redress that balance using reflection on some of John's supervisory experiences (as a supervisee) with Paul (the clinical supervisor) over a 10-month period whilst working as a team clinical supervisor in mental health practice. As the cursor blinks on the laptop and in reviewing our journey, we are reminded that uncertainty is the companion of the reflective practitioner. In particular, for the supervisee who took in issues about his supervisory practice, and for the supervisor, in supporting those reflections and offering an alternative way of seeing CS. More specifically, the chapter has the following aims.

- To demonstrate the processes of reflection and CS as a method of learning for an experienced clinical supervisor.
- To explore some of the key themes arising from our reflections about 'supervision on supervision' that might be relevant to other working clinical supervisors in practice.
- To pose further questions for the ongoing support and development of working clinical supervisors in nursing practice beyond some introductory training.

Making connections between reflective practice and clinical supervision

You might be forgiven for automatically assuming that engaging in CS is a natural extension of reflective practice, and in many ways it is. However, Freshwater (2007, p.51) reminds us that not all authors agree that reflective practice is integral to CS because both concepts have developed independently of each other and have separate, although integrated, theoretical underpinnings. For instance, other chapters in this book attribute the roots of reflection and reflective learning to educational philosophers such as John Dewey (1933), Donald Schön (1983, 1987), Paulo Freire (1972) and the development of professional teaching and education of adult learners (Knowles 1984; Knowles *et al.* 2005), amongst others. Of particular importance in relation to CS is the process of learning *through* experience, or what is often referred to as 'experiential' learning (Kolb 1984). The stages of working through an experience towards more trans-formational learning are often portrayed as being a sequential learning cycle (e.g. Kolb 1984; Dennison and Kirk 1990). Whilst this belies the complex nature of experiential learning, it has contributed to the devel-opment of a number of early cyclical reflective models that can be used by supervisees in preparing for a CS session (Van Ooijen 2003, p.15). Some of these are outlined in Chapter 9 of this book, e.g. Driscoll (1994) and Gibbs *et al.* (1988).

Considering the many definitions for nursing on the process of reflec-tion and its application as reflective practice, and also being mindful that these need to be taken at face value (Bulman 2008, p.5), Clarke and Graham (1996, p.26) have best described for us the 'what' and 'how' of reflective practice.

> 'By engaging in reflection people are usually engaging in a period of thinking in order to examine often complex situations or situations. The period of thinking (reflection) allows the individual to make sense of an experience, perhaps to liken the experience with other similar experiences and to place it in context. Faced with complex decisions thinking it through (reflecting) allows the individual to sep-arate out the various influencing factors and come to a reasoned decision or course of action.'

The 'what' is suggestive of purposeful, or what De Bono (1985, p.11) refers to as 'deliberative' thinking, and the 'how' relates to the process of reflection. Based on the above and other definitions that can be found in this book, becoming reflective has as its main characteristics the ability to:

- stop and find time to explore a significant experience in depth, either alone or with others
- recognise how you felt about that experience at the time
- be willing to gain a deeper understanding of what happened
- evaluate the experience from a different perspective but with an emphasis on identifying learning and working towards actions for improvement.

In relation to clinical practice, taking a critical perspective through reflec-tion means that by doing so, you develop a fuller understanding and per-haps become better equipped to deal with a similar situation again in the future (Thompson and Thompson 2008, p.26). As we will see later in the chapter, this is not unlike some of the key principles of CS.

The notion of supervision *per se* in nursing is not new. It comes in many guises and is perhaps considered by some practitioners (wrongly

Box 6.1   Summary of the main components of supervision activities in healthcare (Based on Driscoll and O'Sullivan 2007, p.6)

- Supervised practice and learning (e.g. mentoring and preceptorship often associated with an element of assessing to improve individual performance)
- Organisational or managerial supervision (e.g. child protection supervision, appraisal, performance reviews and disciplinary meetings focusing on the performance of the individual in relation to organisational objectives)
- Supportive supervision (e.g. clinical supervision, peer support, development coaching, networking, action learning, significant incident reviews and associated with the need to share experiences with others to obtain support to change or act)

in our view), as equating to or being CS itself. Box 6.1 summarises the main components of supervision in healthcare practice available to practitioners based on Driscoll and O'Sullivan (2007, p.6). It could be argued that there is considerable overlap with such a simple classification limiting the range of supervision activities available in clinical practice by placing them into convenient categories. For instance, does organisational supervision mean it is not supportive or that reflection and learning might not occur in all three forms of supervision? Accepting this limitation, what might be more easily recognisable is the distinct intentions behind each of the three supervisory components, not just for those being supervised but in particular for those in a supervisory role. As Heath and Freshwater (2000) rightly assert, supervisory relationships and approaches will differ depending on the intentions of those engaging in them.

Clinical supervision as a practice-based activity has not 'gone away' since its inception (Department of Health 1993) and continues to evolve, albeit slowly, as a predominantly supportive and developmental form of supervision for UK registrant nurses, health visitors and more latterly, support workers from a variety of allied health professions (Royal College of Nursing 2006, p.14). There is an increased organisational and professional legitimacy through ongoing NHS reforms, and in particular Clinical Governance. Clinical Governance remains a central tenet in UK governmental healthcare reforms, providing a statutory quality framework through which all healthcare organisations are accountable for continually improving service delivery (Sale 2005; McSherry and Pearce 2011). In our view, this has dramatically raised the profile of continuing professional development (CPD) and work-based learning activities including CS, in meeting those statutory regulatory requirements. For instance, healthcare in England is regulated in law by the Care Quality Commission (CQC) with similar bodies functioning in the other countries of the United Kingdom. Healthcare organisations (including NHS hospitals) are required to comply and demonstrate evidence through regular inspection and audit against the published standards on the quality of care and safety of residents/patients being delivered (Care Quality Commission 2010). Of the 16 Regulations that come within Part 4 of the Health and Social Care Act (2008), one of those outcomes (Outcome 14c, p.137) relates specifically to staff support and states:

> …staff are supported and managed at all times … a support structure is in place for supervision … staff can talk through any issues about their role, or about the people they provide care, treatment and support to, with their line manager or supervisor …

The implication of this has been that many healthcare providers now have to work towards ensuring that supervisory structures are available to all staff through organisational and managerial support, as well as policy direction. The transferring of supervision policy ideals into the realities of everyday clinical practice still requires a sea change by practitioners to value taking time out for CS as a legitimate form of learning and support, as well as 'doing' the clinical work. Although not mandatory for registrant nurses, engaging in CS is a professional as well as organisational requirement. The Nursing and Midwifery Council (2008), which regulates nursing and midwifery in the UK, states that the principles and relevance of CS should be included in all pre-registration and postregistration education programmes and all registrant nurses should have access to a clinical supervisor. It cites the original NHS Management Executive definition (Department of Health 1993, p.15 para.3.27) as:

> … a formal process of professional support and learning which enables individual practitioners to develop knowledge and competence, assume responsibility for their own practice and enhance consumer protection and safety of care in complex situations. It is central to the process of learning and to the scope of the expansion of practice and should be seen as a means of encouraging self-assessment and analytical and reflective skills …

In many ways, this original definition encompasses the broad range of supervisory activities available to nurses alluded to earlier, but also offers some clues for what supervisees might take into the CS encounter, e.g. the need for support, ways of managing patients (or staff) more effectively, as well as the possibilities for future learning through a process of reflection as self-assessment. Rather than prescribe any particular model, the Nursing and Midwifery Council (2008) makes connections with reflection as a vehicle for CS when it describes one of the six principles as being: '... a practice-focused professional relationship involving a practitioner reflecting on practice guided by a skilled supervisor ...'.

We hasten to add that not all reflection is CS; for instance, reflection can include discussing ways of achieving better grades in a tutorial, gaining feedback from a mentor on handling a complex admission to the ward, or considering alternative ways of communicating to medical colleagues with a preceptor or manager. Fowler and Chevannes (1998) warn that imposing reflection as a model for CS on people for whom that style is inappropriate will lead to avoidance and further implementation challenges. What we believe is that the very act of being engaged in a formalised CS relationship cannot help but *potentiate* reflective practice. We say potentiate, as the term 'reflection' is used so widely in normal parlance that it seems to encapsulate all manner of thinking. More *critical reflection* (in the CS process we engaged in) involves much deeper examination on what we are thinking, our feelings about a practice experience and importantly what learning is taking place to inform future actions. Fook and Gardner (2007, p.51), in their model of critical reflection, go further, stating that the purpose of critical reflection is to intentionally unsettle the dominant thinking of the practitioner within professional practice so it can be reworked through reflection. In this sense, critical reflection is the process that really *potentiates* reflective practice through challenging a practitioner's thinking before its application into the work situation, for instance through altering perspectives, trying something different or recognising that further knowledge or enquiry is required. So whilst all practitioners have the potential to critically reflect on themselves in relation to their practice, it does not necessarily follow that they will, or even wish to. This poses a further challenge to the implementation and acceptance of CS in everyday clinical work.

Specifically in relation to CS, developing the ability to critically reflect is therefore likely to be dependent on a number of factors.

- Knowing what the expectations are for CS
- Knowing who the clinical supervisor is
- A willingness by the supervisee to reflect (and act upon) aspects of the self in practice
- The environment in which critical reflection takes place
- The knowledge and skills of the CS participants in critical reflection
- The ongoing CS relationship

Bond and Holland (2010, p.15) make a significant contribution with their definition of CS that not only describes the process but makes the role of the supervisee and clinical supervisor more explicit.

Chapter 6

Clinical supervision is regular, protected time for facilitated, in-depth reflection on complex issues influencing clinical practice. It aims to enable the supervisee to achieve, sustain and creatively develop a high quality of practice through the means of focused support and development. The supervisee reflects on the part she plays as an individual in the complexities of the events and the quality of practice. This reflection is facilitated by one or more experienced colleagues who have expertise in facilitation and the frequent, ongoing sessions are led by the supervisee's agenda. The process of clinical supervision should continue throughout the person's career, whether they remain in clinical practice or move into management, research or education.

It would seem that effective CS is also dependent on the supervisor being able to facilitate reflection as well as support the supervisee's agenda and concerns to develop effective practice. Such facilitation lends itself to developing the ability to guide reflection within the safety of the supervisory space as part of the repertoire of skills needed by a clinical supervisor. It is also suggested that through the mixture of challenge and support when guiding reflection, a clinical supervisor might also be considered a 'critical friend' (Baguley and Brown 2009) or 'critical companion' (Titchen 2003a,b) to the supervisee.

Finally, as a warning to new clinical supervisors, Duffy (2008) cites Chris Johns (2002) who argues that having no guide at all is superior to having a guide who lacks experience or is untrustworthy.

The need to have confidence in the clinical supervisor arises because critical reflection will often unearth hidden fears and possible weaknesses in one's practice. Such disclosures might initially be viewed as threatening or anxiety provoking by opening up one's practice to scrutiny and critical questioning by others. Some authors have gone further, suggesting that the process of reflection in practice might also be interpreted as a form of practice 'confession' (Gilbert 2001) or a method of covert surveillance by management on practice performance (Cotton 2001). Rolfe and Gardner (2006) counter such concerns, stating that reflective practice, and in particular CS, is concerned mainly with learning about one's practice rather than primarily learning about ourselves. However, it is also argued that learning about oneself through practice is the fundamental nature of experiential learning in CS (Fowler 2011, p.57). Supervision possibilities are also dependent on what knowledge, skills and experience are brought into the CS relationship. Regardless of this, it is doubtful whether CS can be significant (or even happen at all) without an open and trusting CS relationship that begins by agreeing what is to happen. Before outlining our CS experiences, we think it useful to have an understanding of the context in which it was carried out.

Background to team supervision as the focus for supervision on supervisory practice

The context for 'supervision on supervision' was John's work as a consultant for the development of CS to a private sector mental health nursing care home in transition. This had included facilitating how CS was to be organised, together with policy direction and offering one-to-one CS to the manager in achieving a new vision for the nursing home. There began a slow cascade effect with CS in which the manager was supervised by John and in turn supervised the registered nurses and an administrator. The qualified nurses, and a senior support worker, became responsible for the supervision of support workers. When the manager left suddenly, John was asked, as an interim measure, if he would supervise a team of three key staff. These were a deputy nurse manager who was acting up but would become the registered manager, the home administrator and a senior support worker, the latter being responsible for development of the support worker team.

Team supervision differs from group supervision as it involves not just coming together for the purposes of joint supervision, but an interrelated work life outside the group, including the sharing of activities and joint responsibilities (Hawkins and Shohet 2011, p.162). All three individuals – the deputy nurse manager, the home administrator and a senior support worker – were rapidly to become 'the new management team'. This included the prompt agreement of new contracts of employment with the proprietor and increased responsibilities as a team for the day-to-day management of the nursing home. At the time of writing, the home administrator left the organisation and team supervision was disbanded, although evaluated as important with the staff transition. John still offers one-to-one CS with the new home manager and continues with Paul for 'supervision on supervision' for his CS work.

Establishing the relationship for supervision on supervision

The notion of the skilled supervisor has previously been cited as an important component for CS in nursing. Hawkins and Shohet (2011, p.215) suggest the first step to becoming that skilled supervisor is to receive good supervision, as without this the working supervisor lacks a role model or the experience of how beneficial supervision can be in one's professional life. We fully endorse these sentiments and throughout our careers have been fortunate enough to have worked with a mixture of good, as well as not so good role models. Through this process, we have also both developed (and continue to learn about) our styles as working clinical supervisors. Additionally, we would suggest that you get out of CS

> ## Box 6.2   The key characteristics of CS in nursing practice
>
> - A planned and intentional opportunity to reflect on practice as a legitimate form of work-based activity with the intention of improving care delivery
> - Conducted within previously agreed boundaries but one in which a number of methods might be adopted to suit the needs of the supervisee, e.g. one-to-one, group, etc.
> - A confidential process (with exceptions) in which a supervisee is ideally able to choose a supervisor to discuss significant aspects of their practice
> - A regular process of organisational support in addition to those informal and *ad hoc* moments in practice
> - A legitimate form of practice-based learning that can be used as evidence towards continuing professional development by a practitioner
> - The focus is on supervisee concerns and issues about practice
> - Offers continuity and support to a supervisee that begins with talking and discussing practice issues with the purpose of learning about ways of improving practice
> - An ongoing learning process in which clinical supervisors are also supervisees themselves

what you are willing to take into that process, for example commitment to CS with regard to preparation, openness to challenge, honesty and, of course, a willingness to learn and act upon such feedback.

We consider that having the ability to choose one's clinical supervisor as a supervisee is a distinct characteristic of CS (Box 6.2). This also includes working clinical supervisors having the opportunity to be supervisees themselves and to choose an appropriate supervisor, the purpose being to reflect on their clinical work, as well as discussing issues in their supervisory role. However, we also acknowledge that this might not always be possible in every practice arena but is something to strive towards. Further possibilities might be to consider someone who does not work immediately in your practice environment but perhaps within your organisation. Other ways might be to look at your available practice networks, or someone who inspires you within your area of work who may act as a clinical supervisor. Networking within a specialist group or with practitioners who have a similar interest can also be considered a form of group CS (Wright *et al.* 1997) and is discussed in Chapter 4. In all circumstances, we advise informing your line manager of your intended choice as this may open up further opportunities to gain access to a clinical supervisor.

Our own experience began as independent facilitators for a large NHS trust's implementation of CS. This led to us becoming co-facilitators of a 'Train the Trainers' programme for clinical supervisors in which we both shared concerns about the development of clinical supervisors beyond our 3-day supervisor development programme. We continued network-ing through the use of email and telephone and arranged to meet one evening to discuss the possibilities for working together in CS. During that evening, we formed an agreement or contract for CS, as well as this being a social meeting, as we both had vested interests in the ongoing development of CS in practice. Whilst Power (2007, p.53) might argue that our relationship could be construed as one of 'friends', we prefer to think of our CS as being a professional relationship in which we both share similar concerns.

The CS documentation we devised and used, including the contract, can be downloaded from www.supervisionandcoaching.com. The key features of the contract specifically relating to John's intended 'supervi-sion on supervision' (Box 6.3) as a supervisee included his expectation of preparation by Paul as the supervisor and the use of one-to-one CS conducted on the telephone (discussed later). Setting and maintaining boundaries is an essential part of formalising CS and differs from other forms of more informal supervision. In our experience, new clinical super-visors on training programmes can become confident after they have completed the first session (the agreement or contract) because, of all CS sessions, this is the most structured and there are things to do and talk about. The importance of an agreement cannot be overemphasised and yet it is not uncommon (anecdotally) to find both the supervisor and supervisee rushing through setting boundaries in CS in order to 'get to the action'. But taking the time to gain agreement forms an important reference point in which boundaries are set, e.g. on confidentiality and what is to happen in the CS process, and, just as importantly, what to do if these are not being met.

The use of the telephone as a method of clinical supervision

Whilst the telephone remains one of the cheapest and simplest technolo-gies and is already used extensively in many forms of counselling and psy-chotherapy (Rosenfield 1996; Copeland 2003; Sanders 2007), its use does not seem widespread in nursing CS (Driscoll and Townsend 2007, p.144). The use of a ward telephone or personal mobile for a 'quick chat' to help with an issue in practice, not unlike a chance meeting in a corridor, in our view does not constitute CS. However, we acknowledge it can be an essential method of informal support for surviving the everyday realities of practice. Gardner et al. (2010) argue that such dependence on informal support has hindered the development of CS as a formal relationship, leading to superficial supervision. Perhaps not surprisingly, a practitioner with access to such 'instant' support may question the need to find time to engage in a more arduous process of finding a supervisor, preparing for supervision and formally reflecting on aspects of improving their practice.

Box 6.3   Key features of the CS contract made between John and Paul

Frequency/ session duration	Monthly, 60-minute telephone call (maximum)
Method used	One-to-one telephone conversations John to phone Paul at a designated time (evenings after 20.00) Email support/follow-up
Supervisee expectations	External eye on facilitating team supervision Safe space for challenge and support Opportunity to reflect on my own supervision Identify key 'supervision on supervision' issues for intended book chapter Commitment by supervisor to 'meeting' on agreed dates Pre-preparation by supervisor to read CS documentation forwarded prior to each session
Supervisor expectations	Sessions to take place on a Tuesday or Wednesday evening after 20.00 Supervisee comes prepared for the session Supervisee phones on time and if applicable, gives notice to cancel session Use of supervision to help identify supervision on supervision issues Examine some of the processes of supervision Will assist in supervisor studies in counselling supervision
Maintaining confidentiality	Each person accountable for confidentiality to each other Use of email as a supplement to the session
Other issues	Verbal review at the end of each session using 'least and best' questions, e.g. What I liked least/best about today's session Fuller review after completion of four sessions Issues for Paul relating to a new telephone method of facilitating CS Invasion of personal space, e.g. session outside normal working hours

The telephone solved the problem of having to meet face to face on a regular basis and circumnavigated the need for extensive travel. It is also possible to record and play back a telephone conversation for future transcribing and research purposes, as well as providing evidence of CS.

Although this opportunity for transcribing has not yet been taken up, it remains a possibility for our future work together. Some of the obvious benefits of the telephone CS method we found were:

- direct access to a supervisor of choice who was not immediately available in the work setting
- more likely to fit in with busy work schedules
- challenges the insistence of face-to-face encounters as a preferred method of CS
- preparing more thoroughly for sessions, including use of supplementary email
- feelings of being more in control of the supervision environment, including privacy
- greater need to check assumptions on the telephone when four of the five senses are not being used and the voice is the only clue
- improved use of auditory clues for active listening, e.g. voice, tone, use of words to increase understanding
- physical and psychological feelings of being listened to.

Despite these benefits, there are also some practical questions to address in using the telephone method of CS, e.g. how much will it cost and who will call whom? Other practicalities to be overcome include trying to make notes whilst holding the telephone (use of a headset is an obvious solution), ensuring the telephone is free for the timed incoming call and avoiding interruptions (dogs barking!). Also, it seems that more concentration is required when listening to what is being said, as well as not being said. This was particularly the case for us in the evening when our time boundaries became stretched from 60 to 90 minutes and needed to be reviewed.

ACTIVITY

In relation to your own realities compared to ours, what might be some of the opportunities or challenges posed in using the telephone as an optional method of CS?

How appropriate or not might the telephone method be as a form of CS for you in practice?

Using reflection for supervision on (John's) supervision

As we review our sessions for this chapter on CS and consider what will now become the next phase of our work together, John is reminded of Paul's words on the need to be creative in supervision (Lahad 2000; Schuck and Wood 2011); it would also have been helpful to have read Sylvina Tate's chapter in this book before setting out on our journey together!

Rosenberg (2010) suggests that a motivator for reflection can often be the unconscious pursuit of happiness. In relation to clinical practice, a reason for wanting to reflect on an experience might be feeling upset about something that happened. Launer (2003, p.93) continues this theme, suggesting CS is: '... an opportunity for a professional to change a story about a working encounter by holding a conversation with another professional ...'. It is interesting to note that he is a UK general practitioner who promotes a narrative-based approach in primary care supervision with his colleagues. The purpose of using a storytelling approach in CS is to invite change (in the supervisee), in relation to a situation that they perceive may have not gone well.

This was the starting point for John's reflections, in taking to CS issues that he was unhappy about regarding his own work as a clinical supervisor. We were reminded of Atkins and Murphy's (1993) model of reflection in which the first stage is triggered by an awareness of uncomfortable thoughts or feelings (in this case, John's supervision practice when facilitating team supervision). However, this then progresses on to more detailed analysis and opportunity for personal change in supervision through:

- an increased awareness of uncomfortable feelings and thoughts
- critical analysis of feelings and knowledge
- development of new perspectives.

John's feelings and concerns were captured in a learning journal using an adapted 'open-page technique' (Jasper 2008, p.183). The left-hand page described some of his initial thoughts, concerns and challenges about his facilitation of team supervision, leaving the right-hand page for further analysis. This was often filled in as preparation and to gather his thoughts before team supervision took place, and through making notes of what actually happened immediately after the event, sitting in the car. These descriptive jottings formed the basis for further analysis and, more importantly, as preparation for the next CS session with Paul in which he summarised his thoughts in the form of a 'tabloid headline' such as:

- Supervisee Projectile Vomits Over Supervisor
- Merlin the Magician or Piggy in the Middle?
- Who's in charge of CS ... Daddy Bird?

Whilst these will not be significant to you the reader, driving home in the car and constructing a headline through deconstructing what went on helped John to summarise his feelings about the supervisory practice. The ongoing process of reflection in CS might also be evidenced in the way those headlines developed into more specific 'Questions to Address

ONE-TO-ONE TELEPHONE CLINICAL SUPERVISION DOCUMENTATION	
Clinical Supervisee: John Driscoll	Clinical Supervisor: Paul Cassedy
Date of Clinical Supervision:	
REVIEW OF PROGRESS ON ACTION POINTS PREVIOUSLY AGREED:	
ISSUE/TOPIC FOR DISCUSSION THIS TIME (IN THE FORM OF QUESTION(S)):	
WHY THIS IS IMPORTANT TO ME:	
KEY POINTS FROM DISCUSSION WITH SUPERVISOR:	
NOW WHAT? SUPERVISEE ACTIONS NEXT TIME:	NOW WHAT? ACTIONS FOR NEXT TIME: Clinical Supervisor (where appropriate):
ON REFLECTION/EVALUATION: What I liked least about the session/meeting today: What I liked best about the session/meeting today:	ON REFLECTION/EVALUATION: Clinical Supervisor: What I liked least about the session/ meeting today: What I liked best about the session/ meeting today:
Signed: *Clinical Supervisee*	Signed: *Clinical Supervisor*

Figure 6.1 Ongoing CS documentation as a structure for reflection.

Tonight' that were emailed to Paul as preparation for CS. Subsequent supervision notes became the content of more detailed analysis on the right-hand page of the journal. Our CS documentation (Figure 6.1) in itself became a loose structure for reflection when used in conjunction with the learning journal. Looking back at what happened, the discipline of 'capturing' significant experiences with the intention of identifying learning needs as a working clinical supervisor, use of a learning journal and supplementary use of email were the cornerstones (as well as evidence) of our reflective processes in CS.

Focusing on the supervisory process to identify 'blind spots'

McCormack and Henderson (2007, p.109) suggest CS is a mechanism for 'going beyond the obvious', opening up the possibility of exploring deeper aspects of the self. Developing self-awareness is commonly cited as a skill in becoming a reflective practitioner (Atkins and Schutz 2008, p.30) and is the essence of a well-used definition of reflection by Boyd and Fales (1983, p.113): '... the process of internally examining and exploring an issue of concern, triggered by an experience, which creates and clarifies meaning in terms of self and which results in a changed conceptual perspective'.

A key purpose of exploring John's work as a supervisor with Paul was to become more self-aware of what he did in team supervision. Whilst providing an opportunity for personal and professional improvement as a clinical supervisor, it also presented us both with deeper insights about the sorts of issues that might be raised during 'supervision on supervision'.

The use of parallel process

Focusing on the process of what was going on in our virtual CS 'room', on the telephone, with Paul, was like having a mirror held up to what I was like *inside* the team supervision room. This differed significantly from my own reflective approach in which, as a supervisor, I normally centred on learning and working towards actions and outcomes after the event with supervisees. I was reminded of a quote by Kierkegaard, a Danish philosopher (cited by Carroll 2009), who suggests that although life is lived forward, you understand it backwards or through making sense of past experiences. An example of working in the 'process of supervision' relates to my frustration at the team cancelling sessions due to work commitments and wondering whether there was another agenda, e.g. did they want to end team supervision or not want me as their supervisor? As part of their ongoing work as a team, we discussed priorities in time management, including the importance of team supervision as part of their work activities. Speaking to Paul about my concerns, he reminded me of several occasions when I had done the same thing, when cancelling our supervision, e.g. through attendance at my father's funeral, being stuck in Glasgow with no flights because of snow, and an email correspondence I sent about an evening telephone CS meeting:

'Sorry to be a nuisance Paul. Anne's arranged a decorator to come round on 'Wednesday evening' who is unable to commit to a time … I probably won't be interrupted but don't want this at the back of my mind on the night … can you give me a time for another evening?'

This process of 'mirroring' (Dombeck and Brody 1995) or what is also termed a 'parallel process' (Playle and Mullarkey 1998) was identified in my supervision with Paul, in that I was also unconsciously displaying those same characteristics during my facilitation of team supervision. Mattinson (1975, p.11) further defines parallel process in the following terms which was not unlike our supervision together.

'The processes at work currently in the relationship between client and worker (*John and the team supervisees*) are often reflected in the relationship between worker and supervisor (*John and Paul*)'.

A further blind spot identified in John's supervision was his lack of time management when facilitating a team supervision session, when he sometimes violated his CS agreement by running over time. Another parallel process was noticed when reflecting on our own time management in supervision. For instance, we often ran over time on the telephone. In an informal review of our supervision together, Paul also acknowledged how, as my supervisor, *he* had concerns at his own lack of time boundaries, due to this new method of supervision, and doing CS of an evening rather than during work time, although we had agreed to this beforehand.

The highlighting of these examples of parallel processing enhanced my learning and development both as a supervisee and in my team supervision relationship as a supervisor. An unrecognised parallel process can result in an impasse or barriers to the development of the supervision relationship (Playle and Mullarkey 1998) and even the usefulness of supervision itself (Faugier 1992). Recognising parallel processes through focusing on the process of supervision provided a more creative way of enabling me to become more self-aware of my work as a team supervisor and enhanced the supervisory relationship with Paul.

Hawkins and Shohet (2011, p.82) outline two broad approaches in CS from the disciplines of counselling and psychotherapy that highlighted our different ways of working in supervision.

- Looking to the past to see the future (the supervisee's work is discussed and reflected upon in CS –John's favoured approach)
- Looking at the present to see the future (what goes on in CS is an extension of what goes on in the supervisee's practice – Paul's favoured approach).

The first approach lends itself to what Schön (1991) refers to as reflection-on-action in which the supervisee looks back at significant events with the intention of learning from them and developing strategies to improve. The second (Paul's) approach is often referred to as being in the 'here and now' (Hughes and Morcom 1996, p.48) or process-centred supervision.

Reflecting on the process of our supervision, we are both in agreement with Gilbert and Evans (2009, p.1) that supervision is a learning process in which the supervisee engages with a more experienced practitioner for ongoing development, which in turn promotes and safeguards the well-being of those being cared for. Alongside the more common foci of supervision for the supervisee, e.g. reflection on practice, we have also identified the usefulness of recognising unconscious processes and the relational themes that arise from them in both practice situations and the dynamics of supervision. Hawkins and Shohet's (2011) process model and Gilbert and Evans' (2009) integrative relational model are examples of process-centred supervision models, the latter being Paul's approach as a supervisor. Such a 'here and now' process has enabled John's (and Paul's) development and what Playle and Mullarkey (1998) refer to as a much deeper appreciation of uncovering and gaining clues to the emergence of unconscious feelings in supervision. As Paul stated as part of our review of supervision, working creatively in this way meant that the icing on the (supervision) cake was deeper, richer and more fulfilling.

Game playing in supervision

A natural extension of working 'in process' in CS is how unconscious 'games' are played out between the supervisee and supervisor, perhaps mirroring or replaying what happens when a supervisor facilitates CS. Van Ooijen (2003, p.142) describes such 'games' which need to be guarded against, or at least challenged, as part of any ongoing supervision relationship. For example:

- who is the best practitioner? (competitiveness between the supervisee and supervisor)
- my model is better than yours (having different theoretical orientations)
- become my ideal (supervisor wanting the supervisee to conform to his/her vision of the ideal supervisor)
- I have all the answers you need to know (creating dependency or frustration in the supervisee).

In relation to CS, Lynch *et al.* (2008, p.105) state that clinical supervisors should use their own CS as a way of identifying and dealing with their blind spots, which they describe as:

> '... like trying to drive to a destination that is unfamiliar, without directions or resources such as a map; you may think you know what you are doing or where you are going. The risks are numerous: you could run out of petrol, end up in a deserted area, or be very late for an appointment. To minimise the impact you would need to recognise that you did not know where you were driving before you left rather than when you were already lost!'

The metaphor is a good one and reminds us of John's concerns with the dynamics of team supervision where he thought he knew in which direction he was going, but was fortunate not to get totally lost, because of having 'supervision on his supervision' or a rear view mirror! Blind spots refer to those hidden things John was unable to see by himself. Paul, as the supervisor, had the luxury of being at arm's length from John's supervisory practice, without the emotional attachment of being directly involved, hearing about what happened some time after the event(s). In many ways, he had to not only listen to what was said in CS but consider what was *not* being said, a major insight for John. Further supervisory blind spots identified in John's practice that continue to be worked on with Paul relate to:

- the use of humour to deflect criticism
- the burden of being perceived (and hired) as an expert
- raising the bar too high for supervisees to achieve change
- feeling responsible for the behaviour of supervisees
- doing the work of others in supervision
- initial feelings of becoming deskilled when reflecting on supervisory practice.

It is not difficult to imagine how some of those blind spots might also manifest in the supervision room as unconscious games with supervisees, in the absence of any supervision for supervisors.

Supervisory preferences and styles

Navigating the supervision boat is an experiential exercise John devised as part of his training of clinical supervisors. It is based on Brigid Proctor's (1986) functions or elements of CS (Figure 6.2), where an observer notes which one of those main functions the supervisor seems to prefer when working with their supervisee. Having a working knowledge of the three functions can offer direction for a new clinical supervisor to help the

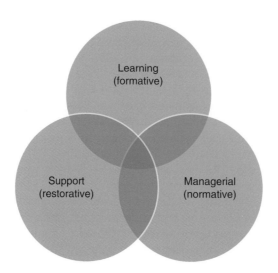

Figure 6.2   Functions of clinical supervision (Based on Proctor 1986).

supervisee explore a story in more depth. What is often missed by the supervisor is asking what we consider to be the fundamental question at the end of the supervisee's description of what happened: '… based on what you have told me so far, what would YOU (as the supervisee) like to be the main focus of your discussion in the time we have today, in relation to what was happening?'. In this way, CS retains as one of its main characteristics that it is the supervisee who navigates the supervision boat (with the help of the supervisor); this differs significantly from more managerial forms of supervision in practice.

A further way in which 'supervision on supervision' supported John as a supervisee is through an increased self-awareness of his own strengths and weaknesses, and further skill development in relation to using each of Proctor's functions when acting as a supervisor. For instance, based on his background in teaching and coaching and his general knowledge of CS and reflective practice, there is an obvious preference when working as a supervisor towards facilitating learning (formative) and support (restorative) with a lower preference for managing (normative). In an ideal situation, the clinical supervisor should be flexible enough to facilitate all three functions. However, team supervision proved a challenge to John's preferences when the supervisees' (and organisational) emphasis appeared to be towards more managerial forms of supervision. This was reflected in the following learning journal headline: *Merlin the Magician or Piggy in the Middle?*. This posed further questions to reflect on in his supervision.

- Am I (John) being too prescriptive in supervision as a clinical supervisor, e.g. taking on their role and responsibilities as 'the expert', or is this as a direct result of wishing to protect the team and not wanting them to fail?

- My feeling is to continue with a more managerial form of supervision with the team for the time being … why am I not willing to consider more facilitative approaches which is my usual style?

An extract in John's learning journal following supervision with Paul revealed the following.

'… I think part of my learning is to be much more guided by the team … perhaps I have been trying too hard with clinical supervision and missed that they might not be working at that level yet, for instance, they have enough to think about with adapting to their new managerial roles … I wonder how willing I have been with the team in altering my own style of supervision to suit their needs?

The concept of supervisory styles, particularly in relation to the training of new clinical supervisors, and the work of John Heron's (1976) six-category intervention analysis (Box 6.4) has some predominance in the UK nursing literature (Cutcliffe and Epling 1997; Sloan and Watson 2002; Sloan 2006, p.64; Sloan 2007, p.105; Bond and Holland 2010, p.157; Cassedy 2010, p.106; Hawkins and Shohet 2011, p.135). Two broad categories of interpersonal intervention, as a clinical supervisor with a supervisee, are authoritative and facilitative. Both of these approaches have three subcategories that became the foci for discussion in supervision. John's concerns were how to develop a more facilitative style with the team, as he was perceived as an expert and employed to act as a clinical supervisor. Bond and Holland (2010, p.131) warn how the learning potential of clinical supervisors can be reduced if they believe that they should have all the answers, present themselves as experts and not disclose any concerns to supervisees about working in CS.

Chapter 6

Box 6.4   Heron's (1976) six-category intervention analysis (Adapted from Heron 1976)

Authoritative interventions	Facilitative interventions
Prescriptive, e.g. giving advice, directing what is to be done	Cathartic, e.g. allowing the release of emotion
Informative, e.g. giving information, instructing	Catalytic, e.g. encouraging reflection through questioning about ways of solving concerns
Confrontative, e.g. being challenging, giving direct feedback	Supportive, e.g. validating and acknowledging what is happening

As a result of this, further work was undertaken by John who carried out a modified form of the Briggs and Briggs-Myers (2000) personality profile online (BSM Consulting 2011). In this he was caricatured as an 'ENFJ' or 'The Giver', best suited to a career in teaching, facilitating and consulting amongst others. Although 'The Giver' is suggested to have a talent for bringing out the best in people and reflected John's personality in supervision, he was minded that sometimes this could lead to (unconsciously) manipulating supervisees to act in a particular way. Smythe (2004) offers a worked example specifically relating to nurse teachers (and John continues to undertake university work), who are often more engrossed in supplying information than in inviting thinking in their students. Further work in supervision has led to John experimenting with silence as an intentional learning strategy in team supervision, or what Bond and Holland (2010, p.224) refer to as facilitating a more 'space-giving mode' in contrast to more directive or collaborative methods as a supervisor.

Just like supervision for supervisors: more questions than answers?

So far, we have illustrated some examples from our own experience of supervision on supervision. In this final section of the chapter, we consider what further questions emerged from our supervision on supervision and broader issues for the development of CS in nursing practice. Like our ongoing efforts illustrated through working together in supervision, our work is incomplete and it is difficult to make any firm inferences for the work of other clinical supervisors in nursing practice.

ACTIVITY

Think about your own support currently received as a working clinical supervisor. Is it of a more formal (like ours) or informal nature? How do you think this might impact on your decision to periodically seek out CS on your supervision?

This exploratory work in supervision on supervision was intentional and based on our concerns for working clinical supervisors. However, inferences *can* be made about John's future supervisory practice. Not unlike the process of reflection itself, surprises such as uncovering his supervisory 'blind spots', even as an experienced clinical supervisor, raised further questions, choices and options. However, uncertainty is the certainty of becoming and being a reflective practitioner. Carroll (2009) goes further, stating that the role of the clinical supervisor to facilitate deeper learning with the supervisee is to *intentionally manufacture* uncertainty in the supervisee's work. Undoubtedly there was evidence of this intention that led not just to a sense of a changed perspective, but willingness to change and act in John's supervisory work. The process has also been an example of collaborative learning through reflection, in which Paul gained further insight into his work as a clinical supervisor and also experienced a new telephone method of facilitating supervision. We are both left with further uncertainty, as two experienced supervisors, about how ethical it is to practise as a clinical supervisor without that same supervisor having access to any periodic supervision on their 'giving' of supervision. It would seem a profound contradiction that a clinical supervisor, however experienced in facilitating reflection in the supervisee(s), might not be prepared to find the time to engage in a similar process of reflection on their 'giving' of supervision.

Supervision on supervision as a distinct characteristic of CS would seem to be the 'icing on the cake', or something that might be applied after CS has been more fully created in and for practice. In our view with process-centred supervision (which ours was), there *is* a need to regularly review what is happening within the supervisory relationship. In more traditional forms of CS that utilise reflection on practice as an approach (e.g. after the event), supervision can perhaps be more periodic or lend itself to reflecting on one's supervisory practice in a facilitated peer group. What is vital is that there is ongoing support and development of working clinical supervisors, beyond some rudimentary training. This has still not been agreed upon in nursing. We suggest that ongoing supervisory support should include policy direction to enhance the opportunity for supervision on supervision: this is an essential ingredient for CS to be sustained in practice.

It might be argued that both authors have a vested interest in the development of CS, and have demonstrated a willingness to explore the notion of supervision on supervision by openly engaging in the process, in addition to the everyday work we do. We wonder whether in your own experience you consider CS to be an everyday work-related activity and a method of staff support, or whether it can only be realised in your own time. It would seem critical (perhaps even obvious) for the development of ever transforming health services, increased expectations for delivering quality services and further demands on practitioners, that time is found to STOP to think critically about nursing practice.

In this chapter we now raise further questions not just about what happens in the supervision room but the quality of supervision being offered. Once again, we state that supervision on supervision, which might be regarded by some as the 'icing on the CS cake', is an essential element of the overall development of CS in practice.

This chapter demonstrates a fusion of two different forms of reflection leading to what we feel has been a more reflective supervisory practice, one in which the focus (and expertise of the supervisor) has been to examine what happens in the 'here and now' to inform future supervisory practice. The other has been to 'look at the past' (and expertise of the supervisee) to inform future supervisory practice. One of the insights from reflecting on our supervision on supervision together has been to indirectly address the question: *How have I become the clinical supervisor I am, but also now wish to become*? Nicholls (2007, p.86) reminds us of the importance of letting our questions stand in CS and not to rush to conclusions. What he meant was that often, the questions being posed, as in this chapter, are our questions as authors and supervisors but may not be your questions as the reader. So, rather than make a definitive conclusion, we prefer to pose further questions arising from our own reflective experiences. They are not intended to be an exhaustive list or placed in any particular order. However, we envisage that such questions will stimulate professional debate about whether supervision on supervision for supervisors is either necessary or desirable.

- What evidence supports the notion that periodic supervision on supervision is happening in nursing practice?
- What evidence supports the idea that having supervision on supervision leads to more effective work as a clinical supervisor?
- Where do clinical supervisors currently go for support as working clinical supervisors?
- How ethical is it to practise as a clinical supervisor with others without being part of the process oneself?
- What are the likely outcomes if there is no CS or active support for working clinical supervisors in practice?
- In what ways might CS be considered ineffective or even harmful in unskilled hands?
- What do I do if I get 'stuck' working as a new (or experienced) clinical supervisor in practice?
- What might be the stages of development for a working clinical supervisor beyond a rudimentary training programme?
- What is the professional view on the work of clinical supervisors being regulated in the future?
- In what ways might the development of professional guidelines be helpful to the clinical supervisor in CS?
- What professional and organisational policy support exists for the ongoing development of working clinical supervisors?

Acknowledgements

Our personal thanks go to Chris Bulman for her support and giving us the opportunity to share some of our supervisory concerns to a wider audience. Also to the team of supervisees who will know who they are and contributed to the debate. Finally, to the late John Driscoll (senior), who didn't get to see the fruits of this chapter.

References

Arvidsson, B. and Fridlund, B. (2005) Factors influencing nurse supervisor competence: a critical incident analysis study. *Journal of Nursing Management*, **13**(3), 231–237.

Atkins, S. and Murphy, K. (1993) Reflection: a review of the literature. *Journal of Advanced Nursing*, **18**(8), 1188–1192.

Atkins, S. and Schutz, S. (2008) Developing the skills for reflective practice. In: Bulman, C. and Schutz, S. (eds) *Reflective Practice in Nursing*, 4th edn. Wiley-Blackwell, Oxford.

Baguley, M. and Brown, A. (2009) Critical friends: an investigation of shared narrative practice between education and nursing graduates. *Teaching in Higher Education*, **14**(2), 195–207.

Bond, M. and Holland, S. (2010) *Skills of Clinical Supervision for Nurses*, 2nd edn. Open University/ McGraw-Hill Education, Maidenhead.

Boyd, E. and Fales, A. (1983) Reflecting learning: key to learning from experience. *Journal of Humanistic Psychology*, **23**(2), 99–117.

BSM Consulting (2011) The Personality Type Portraits. www.personalitypage. com/html/portraits.html

Bulman, C. (2008) An introduction to reflection. In: Bulman, C. and Schutz, S. (eds) *Reflective Practice in Nursing*, 4th edn. Wiley-Blackwell, Oxford.

Care Quality Commission (2010) *Guidance about Compliance: Essential Standards of Quality And Safety*. Care Quality Commission, London.

Carroll, M. (2009) Supervision: critical reflection for transformational learning. *Clinical Supervisor*, **28**(2), 210–220.

Cassedy, P. (2010) *First Steps in Clinical Supervision: A Guide for Healthcare Professionals*. Open University/ McGraw-Hill Education, Maidenhead.

Clarke, D.J. and Graham, M. (1996) Reflective practice, the use of diaries by experienced registered nurses. *Nursing Review*, **15**(1), 26–29.

Copeland, S. (2003) Supervising on the telephone – stop-gap solution or effective time management? *Counselling and Psychotherapy Journal*, **October**, 34–36.

Cotton, A.H. (2001) Private thoughts in public spheres: issues in reflection and reflective practices in nursing. *Journal of Advanced Nursing*, **36**(4), 512–519.

Cutcliffe, J.R. and Epling, M. (1997) An exploration of the use of John Heron's confronting interventions in clinical supervision: case studies from practice. *Psychiatric Care*, **4**, 174–180.

De Bono, E. (1985) *Six Thinking Hats*. Viking Penguin, New York.

Dennison, B. and Kirk, R. (1990) *Do, Review, Learn, Apply: A Simple Guide to Experiential Learning*. Blackwell Education, Oxford.

Department of Health (1993) *Vision for the Future: The Nursing, Midwifery and Health Visiting Contribution to Health and Health Care*. Department of Health, London.

Dewey, J. (1933) *How We Think: A Restatement of the Relation of Reflective Thinking to the Educative Process*. D.C. Heath, Boston.

Dombeck, M. and Brody, S. (1995) Clinical supervision: a three-way mirror. *Archives of Psychiatric Nursing*, **9**(1), 3–10.

Driscoll, J.J. (1994) Reflective practice for practice – a framework of structured reflection for clinical areas. *Senior Nurse*, **14**(1), 47–50.

Driscoll, J. and O'Sullivan, J. (2007) The place of clinical supervision in modern healthcare. In: Driscoll, J.J. (ed) *Practising Clinical Supervision: A Reflective Approach*, 2nd edn. Baillière Tindall/Elsevier, Edinburgh.

Driscoll, J. and Townsend, A. Alternative methods in clinical supervision: beyond the face-to-face encounter. In: Driscoll, J.J. (ed) *Practising Clinical Supervision: A Reflective Approach*, 2nd edn. Baillière Tindall/Elsevier, Edinburgh.

Duffy, A. (2008) Guided reflection: a discussion of the essential components. *British Journal of Nursing*, **17**(5), 334–339.

Faugier, J. (1992) The supervision relationship. In: Butterworth, T. and Faugier, J. (eds) *Clinical Supervision in Mentorship and Nursing*. Chapman and Hall, London.

Fook, J. and Gardner, F. (2007) *Practising Critical Reflection: A Resource Handbook*. Open University/ McGraw-Hill Education, Maidenhead.

Fowler, J. (2011) Experiential learning: an underpinning theoretical perspective for clinical supervision. In: Cutcliffe, J.R., Hyrkas, K. and Fowler, J. (eds) *Routledge Handbook of Clinical Supervision. Fundamental International Themes*. Routledge, Abingdon.

Fowler, J. and Chevannes, M. (1998) Evaluating the efficacy of reflective practice within the context of clinical supervision. *Journal of Advanced Nursing*, **27**(2), 379–382.

Freire, P. (1972) *Pedagogy of the Oppressed*. Herder and Herder, New York.

Freshwater, D. (2007) Reflective practice and clinical supervision: two sides of the same coin? In: Bishop, V. (ed) *Clinical Supervision in Practice: Some Questions, Answers and Guidelines for Professionals in Health and Social Care*, 2nd edn. Palgrave Macmillan, Basingstoke.

Gardner, A., McCutcheon, H. and Fedoruk, M. (2010) Superficial supervision: are we placing clinicians and clients at risk? *Contemporary Nurse*, **34**(2), 258–266.

Gibbs, G., Farmer, B. and Eastcott, D. (1988) *Learning by Doing: A Guide to Teaching and Learning Methods*. Far Eastern University, Birmingham Polytechnic.

Gilbert, M. and Evans, K. (2009) *Psychotherapy Supervision: An Integrative Rational Approach*. Open University Press/McGraw-Hill Education, Maidenhead.

Gilbert T. (2001) Reflective practice and clinical supervision: meticulous rituals of the confessional. *Journal of Advanced Nursing*, **36**(2), 199–205.

Hawkins, P. and Shohet, R. (2011) *Supervision in the Helping Professions*, 3rd edn. Open University/McGraw-Hill Education, Maidenhead.

Heath, H. and Freshwater, D. (2000) Clinical supervision as an emancipatory process: avoiding inappropriate intent. *Journal of Advanced Nursing*, **32**(5), 1298–1306.

Heron, J. (1976) A six-category intervention analysis. *British Journal of Guidance and Counselling*, **4**(2), 143–155.

Hughes, R. and Morcom, C. (1996) *Clinical Supervision – Distance Learning Package*. Warrington Community Health Care Trust, Warrington.

Jasper, M. (2008) Using reflective journals and diaries to enhance practice and learning. In: Bulman, C. and Schutz, S. (eds) *Reflective Practice in Nursing*, 4th edn. Wiley-Blackwell, Oxford.

Johns, C. (2002) *Guided Reflection: Advancing Practice*. Blackwell Science, London.

Knowles, M. (1984) *Andragogy in Action*. Jossey-Bass, San Francisco.

Chapter 6

Knowles, M., Holton, E. and Swanson, R. (2005) *The Adult Learner: A Neglected Species*, 6th edn. Elsevier, London.

Kolb, D. (1984) *Experiential Learning: Experience as the Source of Learning and Development*. Prentice Hall, Englewood Cliffs, New Jersey.

Lahad, M. (2000) *Creative Supervision: The Use of Expressive Arts Methods in Supervision and Self-Supervision*. Jessica Kingsley, London.

Launer, J. (2003) A narrative-based approach to primary care supervision. In: Burton, J. and Launer, J. (eds) *Supervision and Support in Primary Care*. Radcliffe Medical Press, Oxford.

Lynch, L., Hancox, K., Happell, B. and Parker, J. (2008) *Clinical Supervision for Nurses*. Wiley-Blackwell, Chichester.

Mattinson, J. (1975) *The Reflective Process in Casework Supervision*. Tavistock Institute for Marital Studies, London.

McCormack, B. and Henderson, L. (2007) Critical reflection and clinical supervision: facilitating transformation. In: Bishop, V. (ed) *Clinical Supervision in Practice: Some Questions, Answers And Guidelines For Professionals in Health and Social Care*, 2nd edn. Palgrave Macmillan, Basingstoke.

McSherry, R. and Pearce, P. (2011) *Clinical Governance: A Guide to Implementation for Healthcare Professionals*, 3rd edn. Wiley-Blackwell, Chichester.

Milne, D. (2009) *Evidence-Based Clinical Supervision: Principles and Practice*. British Psychological Society/John Wiley, Chichester.

Nicholls, D. (2007) Essential elements for a successful supervisory partnership to flourish. In: Driscoll, J.J. (ed) *Practising Clinical Supervision: A Reflective Approach*, 2nd edn. Baillière Tindall/Elsevier, Edinburgh.

Nursing and Midwifery Council (2008) *Clinical Supervision for Registered Nurses*. Nursing and Midwifery Council, London.

Playle, J. and Mullarkey, K. (1998) Parallel process in clinical supervision: enhancing learning and providing support. *Nurse Education Today*, **18**(7), 558–566.

Power, S. (2007) Boundaries and responsibilities in clinical supervision. In: Driscoll, J.J. (ed) *Practising Clinical Supervision: A Reflective Approach*, 2nd edn. Baillière Tindall/Elsevier, Edinburgh.

Proctor, B. (1986) Supervision: a co-operative exercise in accountability. In: Marken, M. and Payne, M. (eds) *Enabling and Ensuring: Supervision in Practice*. National Youth Bureau, Council for Education and Training in Youth and Community Work, Leicester.

Rolfe, G. and Gardner, L. (2006) Do not ask who I am…: confession, emancipation and (self)-management through reflection. *Journal of Nursing Management*, **14**(8), 593–600.

Rosenberg, L.R. (2010) Transforming leadership: reflective practice and the enhancement of happiness. *Reflective Practice*, **11**(1): 9–18.

Rosenfield, M. (1996) *Counselling by Telephone*. Professional Skills for Counsellors Series. Sage Publications, London.

Royal College of Nursing (2006) *Supervision, Accountability and Delegation of Activities to Support Workers: A Guide for Registered Practitioners and Support Workers*. Intercollegiate information paper developed by the Chartered Society of Physiotherapy, Royal College of Speech and Language Therapists, British Dietetic Association and the Royal College of Nursing. Royal College of Nursing, London.

Chapter 6

Sale, D. (2005) *Understanding Clinical Governance and Quality Assurance: Making it Happen*. Palgrave Macmillan, Basingstoke.

Sanders, P. (2007) *Using Counselling Skills on the Telephone and in Computer Mediated Communication*, 3rd edn. PCCS Books, Ross-on-Wye.

Schön, D. (1983) *The Reflective Practitioner: How Professionals Think in Action*. Basic Books, San Francisco.

Schön, D. (1987) *Educating the Reflective Practitioner*. Jossey-Bass, San Francisco.

Schön, D. (1991) *The Reflective Practitioner: How Professionals Think in Action*. Ashgate Publishing, Aldershot.

Schuck, C. and Wood, J. (2011) *Inspiring Creative Supervision*. Jessica Kingsley, London.

Sloan, G. (2006) *Clinical Supervision in Mental Health Nursing*. Wiley-Blackwell, Chichester.

Sloan, G. (2007) Psychological approaches to the clinical supervision encounter. In: Driscoll, J.J. (ed) *Practising Clinical Supervision: A Reflective Approach*, 2nd edn. Baillière Tindall/Elsevier, Edinburgh.

Sloan, G. and Watson, H. (2002) Clinical supervision models for nursing: structure, research and limitations. *Nursing Standard*, **17**(4), 41–46.

Smythe, E.A. (2004) Thinking. *Nurse Education Today*, **24**(4): 327–332.

Thompson, S. and Thompson, N. (2008) *The Critically Reflective Practitioner*. Palgrave Macmillan, Basingstoke.

Titchen, A. (2003a) Critical companionship: Part 1. *Nursing Standard*, **18**(9), 33–40.

Titchen, A. (2003b) Critical companionship: Part 2 Using the framework. *Nursing Standard*, **18**(10), 33–38.

Van Ooijen, E. (2003) *Clinical Supervision Made Easy*. Churchill Livingstone/Elsevier Science, Edinburgh.

Williams, L. and Irvine, F. (2009) How can the clinical supervisor role be facilitated in nursing: a phenomenological exploration. *Journal of Nursing Management*, **17**(4), 474–483.

Wright, S., Elliott, M. and Scholefield, H. (1997) A networking approach to clinical supervision. *Nursing Standard*, **11**(18), 39–41.

Chapter 7

A personal exploration of reflective and clinical expertise

Sue Duke

Faculty of Health Sciences, University of Southampton, Southampton, UK

Back to the beginning

I remember sitting in the postgraduate centre at the John Radcliffe Hospital, one evening after a seminar, discussing the conception of the first edition of this book. The discussion was charged with passion, purpose and persuasion. I was excited by the possibility of having the opportunity to tell our experience of working with postregistration students, and of the emotional and ethical consequences of reflection we had experienced (as we went on to do in the first edition) (Duke and Copp 1994), and apprehensive about whether I was up to the job. This emotional mixture of excitement and anxiety has been present as I have written for each of the previous editions of this book.

However, this time it has been different; no excitement and good doses of dread. In part, I think this is because those heady days of the early 1990s, when I was lucky enough to be part of a community of very talented practitioners who lived and breathed reflection, are long gone. I find that being reflective – doing reflection – is a big 'ask'. In a clinical world that has become increasingly devoid of resources, increasingly complex in both illness and human terms and increasingly volatile politically, I find reflection increasingly intellectually and emotionally taxing. My apprehension is therefore also to do with feeling somewhat of an imposter in claiming that I might have anything to say about reflection and expert practice.

It is this 'ask' of 'doing reflection' that is central to my experience of writing this chapter. If I am to avoid being an imposter then I need to represent reflection in the current context of healthcare (or my current experience of healthcare) honestly, to not fall into the danger of being idealistic; I need to depict reflection in a real, lived way. This means that revising the chapter I wrote for the previous edition of this book or

Reflective Practice in Nursing, Fifth Edition. Edited by Chris Bulman and Sue Schutz.
© 2013 John Wiley & Sons, Ltd. Published 2013 by John Wiley & Sons, Ltd.

selecting a couple of pre-existing accounts of my practice is not an option, because they do not attend to the current healthcare context or my changing experience with reflection. In addition, to do so would use my reflective accounts as a means to an end, manipulated to mean some-thing that they might not have meant at the time they were experienced and potentially stripped of the sensuality of practice that was associated with the original experience (Duke 2008).

So I need to bite the bullet and embrace the difficulty I am experiencing with being reflective; take Boud *et al.*'s (1985) advice and return to what is within my experience, to help me learn what it is that I want to say about these different reflective times. This chapter therefore starts with a newly written account of my clinical experience, selected because the feelings experienced in the practice mirrored the feeling of dread experienced by the thought of writing this chapter. This reflection is then analysed follow-ing Boud *et al.*'s reflective process: return to the experience, attend to feelings and re-evaluate the experience. I draw upon other exemplars of my reflection and the chapters I have written for previous editions of this book, where they help to illustrate the points I am raising.

Step 1 Return to the experience: finding what is at the heart of your experience

Finding Edna

Edna is an older person whom I went to see in my role as a nurse consult-ant in palliative care with a hospital palliative care team. We had been asked to see Edna to help the ward team with her pain.

The first thing that strikes me when I go into Edna's room is the stark-ness of the room. There is very little in it, a chair with a spare blanket on the seat, a locker with a box of tissues and a side table on which there is a jug of water and observation charts. Edna is curled up in the bed, tiny and barely visible, hidden underneath a sheet, glimpses of a pale night-dress around her neck.

There are no cards on the off-white walls. The blinds at the window are obscuring any view on the outside world and reducing the light entering the room. There are no clues in the room to help me know Edna, just this blank, dark and somewhat empty space.

In contrast, when I go around the bed to the side that Edna is facing and kneel down beside her, take her hand and introduce myself, Edna's face comes alive and I soon find that she has a spirited personality, a quick intellect and honed interpersonal skills. She tells me that she was admit-ted to hospital 4 weeks ago with abdominal pain and that the doctors have been doing tests ever since to find out what is causing this pain. She tells me that she knows that this means bad news and is just waiting to hear exactly what kind of bad news – the doctor has told her that the final tests will be back that morning. We talk a bit about this – what is of most concern to her – being pain free and ensuring that her family are supported. We talk about her family – she is close to her children and their families, does not want to worry them unnecessarily and has found watching their concern mount, as the time has increased without any answers, difficult. We talk about her pain – persistent immobilising abdominal pain occasionally associated with severe cramping pain, helped a bit by the analgesics being given and by keeping still in bed. We talk about sleep and rest – sleep interrupted by pain and worry for her family, rest grabbed between pain during the day.

Finding a diagnosis

As we talk, the surgical registrar comes in and I introduce myself. Edna asks me to stay. He goes around the bed, sits by the side of Edna and explains to her that the tests have confirmed that she has cancer, that surgery is not a possibility to treat this kind of cancer and that he has asked the oncology team to come and see her. He checks that Edna has understood what he has said, and offers to talk to her family if this would be helpful to her. I am deeply impressed by the way that this doctor has compassionately and clearly communicated this news to Edna, by the gentle pace of his conversation and the way that he answered her questions and his concern for her family.

After the registrar leaves, I sit with Edna for a bit (2 or 3 minutes) and then we talk about this conversation a little – it is what she had expected, she is relieved to now have this confirmed, she will take the doctor up on his offer to explain the situation to her children. I move the conversation on to her comfort – explaining that part of our role is to help support her family and that we can return to this conversation to see how best we can do this – but that in the meantime there are some things that we can do for her comfort, which we briefly discuss. I explain that I would like to discuss these with her doctor before he goes off the ward. As I leave her room, I promise to come back shortly to discuss what might be possible.

Finding care

I find the registrar outside Edna's room, discussing the case with the other members of the medical team. The ward staff nurse is nearby but not involved in this conversation. I go and tell her what has just happened and explain that I am going to discuss Edna's comfort with the team and suggest she joins me. The registrar asks me what I think we should do – first I tell him what I found impressive about his conversation with Edna. He is a bit taken aback – he says he is not often offered feedback but then accepts it, pleased and relieved. We make a plan for Edna's pain management, some changes to her regimen to ensure that she has regular continuous morphine for her abdominal pain and some medication available in case this is insufficient to prevent the irregular cramping pain. I am deeply impressed with the staff nurse's confidence with this plan and her speed in finding a colleague to put it into action.

I return to Edna's room and explain what we are planning to do. I check that Edna is happy with this plan – she is – and whether she has any concerns about the change from having morphine now and again to having it regularly – she doesn't, she is just relieved that it might be possible for her pain to be controlled more effectively. As I am beginning to close my conversation with Edna, the staff nurse comes in to give Edna some medication. I leave them, with a plan to come back later.

Family finding me

I am caught on the way out of the ward by Edna's son. He saw me arrive on the ward and go into see his mum and so went off to get some things that she needed from the hospital shop. My first reaction is to be a bit concerned – I have not asked Edna if it would be OK to talk to her family about what has been discussed – her diagnosis and the plans for her comfort and care – and I am also concerned that it might be too soon to do so given that she has only just been told, had not time to think about it, and been in pain. He explains that he went to the shop because he could see that Edna was OK with me for a while, thanks me for showing her respect, explains that he knows that the doctor has seen her and that he is not going to ask me anything to do with this conversation – he says he knows his mum will tell him what she wants him to know. He was just concerned about her comfort and whether I thought we could do anything to help her pain. I explain that we have talked this through, made a plan and that the ward team are beginning to put this in place. I also explain that I am planning to come back later to check that the plan is working but that I anticipated that his mum would be much more comfortable by then.

Side-step: the art of finding knowledge in experience

In my opinion, reflective analysis is the most important part of being reflective because it is central to turning a description of practice into knowledge about practice. Others think so too. For example, Cristicos (1993, p.161), drawing on the work of Aitchison and Graham (1989), suggests that accounts of practice need to be 'arrested, examined, analysed, considered and negated' in order to make the shift from a description of experience to the articulation of practice knowledge. In addition, this work needs to create and clarify meanings 'in terms of self' (Boyd and Fales 1983, p.100) – in other words, in terms of who I am as a practitioner. Furthermore, it is within and through analysis that the potential for reflection to transform practice is initiated (Rolfe 2005).

Finding knowledge in experience in education practice

Before going onto talk about the processes I use to analyse my practice experience, I want to take a slight diversion to draw some inferences from this opinion for educational practice. To me, there is something really important about valuing the place of a careful description of practice and the process of analysing practice in educational practice.

Very often I find in my education practice that students are asked to draw on their experience of practice in their academic work but they are asked to summarise this experience in a small number of words, otherwise they are criticised for being descriptive. I understand the thinking of this guidance – the ability to get to the nub of the matter is an important professional and academic skill.

However, the ability to describe practice is also an important professional skill. If the description of practice is not valued then students are likely to avoid writing descriptions of their practice (there is no need to do so if all that is needed is a short summary) and do not then have the opportunity to hone the skills of crafting an account of practice. Furthermore, if students are not encouraged to develop the ability to describe practice, they do not have access to the texts (their texts) needed to analyse (their) practice. If they do not have texts of practice, they do not learn how to analyse practice and as a consequence they guess what is of importance in a practice experience and need to rely on other kinds of texts (research and theory) to learn about practice or themselves as a practitioner. Thus, their learning about practice is incomplete and biased towards empirical sources. Their professional development is incomplete and potentially biased towards a lack of self-engagement.

I worry that this is a subtle and dangerous form of oppression that stifles our practice voice and suffocates what is at the heart of nursing. The reflective poem in Box 7.1 captures some of my concerns, but it needs to be read on the understanding that it was written one day when I was feeling overwhelmed and isolated by the educational difficulties of encouraging learning from practice. On the whole, we do a good job – we have a rich values-based curriculum and students have dedicated time to learn to become reflective in small learning groups but we need to ensure that students are offered the opportunity to write and analyse reflective texts as well, not just talk reflectively, otherwise written reflective texts will not be sufficiently valued.

Finding the point: start with the text

I use a number of processes to achieve an examination and analysis of my reflective accounts. Working through a process methodically ensures that I uncover the knowledge that is embedded in the account and helps me to engage with what is being revealed. As a consequence, I come to more richly understand my practice and myself as a practitioner.

Box 7.1   Find the point – have a heart: a reflective poem of a recent education experience

I witness,
(in the postgraduate students with whom I work),
confusion and anxiety
when I suggest they write descriptively:
'We've always been told to avoid being descriptive',
I know you have, but that's the point;
when I suggest they start with their practice in an inquiry:
'but what if I cannot find any evidence to support what I want to look at?'
You will and that's the point.
'Well, how many references do you want?'
Reference to you and that's the point.
'Is it OK to use the first person?'
You need to and that's the point.

I witness shock,
when I point out to them the richness and power
in their classroom accounts of practice:
'Oh, I didn't think about it like that'
Well, if you can start to, you'll find the point.
Or they play down the significance
of their practice accounts:
'Well, I suspect we all have examples like this.'
Yes, we do, and that's the point.

I witness reluctance
when I suggest they write this experience
to generate a text for the basis of their assignments:
'But this is just my practice experience,
It's not academic enough for an assignment.'
It can be, and that's the point.

I witness their struggle
with finding their voice
'I think it would be easier to do a more traditional kind of assignment.'
Yes, it would, and that's the point;
with finding the way:
'Can you tell me how to do it?'
It has to be your way, and that's the point.
I listen to their reactions,
after I have read out my reflective analyses in class:
'I will never be able to write anything like that!'
Find your voice, that's the point.

Contd.

I suffer the consequences
of taking this road:
'*What a shame you didn't do a normal PhD, Sue.*'
No, I didn't, but I chose that to be the point.
I listen to students
who are on the receiving end of similar comments:
'*Practice inquiry is not real research,*
better you do an evidence-based practice dissertation.'
Well, you could, but what would be the point?

Let's find the point.
Let's put our hearts back into education.

However, when I first started to write about my experience, I found that the account by itself was sufficient to tell me something about my practice. There was something intrinsically important about crafting an account of an experience; this process made explicit the artistry and process of practice. I also found reading about my practice powerful. I was often struck by the human cost involved in illness and nursing and overwhelmed by the vicarious experience the accounts provoked; how they propelled me into reliving the experience. I illustrated this in an earlier edition with one of the first written accounts of my practice (Duke 2000). I wrote at the end of a shift on an inpatient ward (at the time I was a lecturer practitioner in palliative care): 'Nursed a patient tired of fighting, feeling hopeless. I stayed with the patient but my heart emptied of anything that could protect me' (18/9/91).

When I re-read that entry sometime later, I was struck by the emotion I had caught in the second sentence. This conveyed something I often feel in practice: that nursing requires us to open up our hearts to other people's experience, whole-heartedly, unreservedly. These kinds of reactions often halted any reflective analysis about the practice I had written about. I felt that there was a kind of sacred quality to the accounts (Duke 2007), I guess because they conveyed what is sacred within nursing, the use of self to help another. Whatever the reason, the perception that they were sacred, and that labelling them as sacred, made me feel I did not want to 'mess with them' by pulling them apart – something that would be needed in the process of analysis. In effect, I was 'stunned into silence', paralysed by my emotional and spiritual reaction to the accounts (Duke 2000, p.152).

Finding the point: listen to your emotional response

So my message about the first step of analysis is to pay attention to the emotional reaction that is generated by re-reading the account. If the account is adequately capturing practice experience, it will transmit the sensuality of practice and generate a vicarious emotional response. I take note of this response; it tells me something about the experience that may have been unknown to me at the time, and this generally frees my mind from the paralysis I might otherwise experience.

Finding the point: preserve the wholeness of the text

My second message is that I find that I can move beyond being stunned by preserving the wholeness of the text (respecting the sacredness of the text). I therefore tend to use processes that keep the order of the words intact and rarely summarise the text in any way (Duke 2004, 2008). I also find that seeing what I have written in a visually different way helps me to understand the text differently – to be able to consider other ways of understanding the experience. I therefore tend to follow a process designed by Crepeau (2000). This involves separating the account up into phrases by inserting a hard return on the end of each phrase so that each phrase takes up one line. I then go through the whole text and delete words that do not add anything to the body of the phrase. Thus the first couple of lines of the reflective account above would be transformed as follows:

> *The first thing that strikes me*
> *is the starkness of the room.*
> *There is very little in it,*
> *a chair with a spare blanket*
> *a locker with a box of tissues*
> *a side table with jug of water and charts.*

I then organise the lines into stanzas. Some authors do this by reorganising the order of phrases, juxtaposing those with similar themes to form a stanza (Glesne 1997; Carr 2003). However, I kept the order of the original prose, firstly because I want to keep the order of the text intact, as described above, but also because I have found that the inherent structure of reflective accounts provides a logic that naturally determines the stanzas. I then label each stanza with the idea expressed in that group of phrases. For example, the excerpt above is a complete stanza that I labelled 'first impressions'. At this stage the format of the text becomes what some authors call 'found poetry' (Richardson 2000), text that captures the voice, rhythms and pace of the experience described. The reflective poem in Box 7.1 is an example of a complete piece of reflection that was transformed to a 'found poem' by this process.

Finding the point: find what's in the text

My next step is then to go through the text, slowly and carefully, line by line, and ask questions of the text relating to the reflective cycle. I tend to use the following questions, taken from a synthesis of literature describing reflective processes (Duke and Appleton 2000), because this synthesis is familiar to me, but the questions that others such as Johns (2000) and Fook and Gardner (2007) raise will work equally well.

- What feelings were provoked by this experience?
- What are the salient features here?
- What artistry is being demonstrated?
- What empirical knowledge is being drawn upon?
- What are the ethics of this encounter?
- What personal knowledge am I using?
- How is the context influential?

My next step is to look for the kinds of ways in which I have expressed my practice – for narrative devices. Narrative devices include metaphors and analogies or the use of symbols and images, comparisons or paradoxes, and the choice and way in which words are used, for example through repetition or emphasis.

For example, I use the narrative device of comparison to highlight the difference between the starkness of her room and the richness of her personality:

> *The first thing that strikes me*
> *is the starkness of the room.*
>
> *In contrast...*
> *I quickly find*
> *a spirited personality...*

I use the narrative device of repetition when I am describing the assessment process that I led Edna through:

> *We talk about*
> *what is of most concern to her...*
>
> *We talk about*
> *her family...*
>
> *We talk about*
> *her pain...*
>
> *We talk about*
> *sleep and rest...*

The repetition emphasises what is of importance, in terms of what can be gathered together to generate an understanding of what is important – family, pain, sleep and rest, and what is of importance in how this information is gathered (assessment as talk, conversation).

Box 7.2   Vampires, pirates and aliens

Vampires suck my blood
And wait for me to turn,
Like them, competitive.
I strive to stay alive,
Resist the fanged club,
Instead, collaborate.

Pirates treat me as role
Contender, trespasser,
Accuse me of plunder.
I am no skills thief, but
See red Jolly Rogers
Warning, Hold no quarter!

Aliens baffle me
Their culture quite unique.
We find no meeting space
In which to hold debate
And, instead, like planets
Spin in sep'rate orbit.

The sociologists
Tell me that these three villains
Have other names instead.
Tell how professionals
Keep strangers out, double
Closure I read about.

The dangers of these foes
Include demarcation
and peer separation,
designed to increase power
between colleagues,
but create enemies.

Vampires, pirates, aliens
Symbolic experience
Remind me to value
the nurse in consultancy.
Warn me not to oppress
Others or indoctrinate.

There are no examples of metaphors and analogies in this account, but I quite often use them when I am trying to make sense of something or to say something that feels wrong to say in straightforward prose. For example, the poem 'Vampires, pirates and aliens' (Duke 2007) tells the experience of finding my place as a nurse consultant in an acute hospital and the response of other colleagues to this role (Box 7.2). Shaping this experience by using analogies helped me to depict the experience without it being critical of any particular person or discipline. Using a poetic form to write this experience helped me to be succinct through the discipline of the form (the number of syllables for each line, the number of lines for each verse, the order of words to achieve some rhyme and off-rhyme).

Finding the point: put the story together

Once I have worked through these analytical processes, I usually have a list of thoughts or questions to myself that are more like headings than detailed understandings of the experience. Sometimes a heading will jump out at me, and compel me to go and look at an issue through reference to research and theory. At other times, as with the analysis for this chapter, I am not sure how these thoughts and questions fit together or what kinds of understandings I might draw from them. In this case, I might try and construct a storyline from the thoughts, putting one heading on one sheet of paper or Post-It note and moving the headings around in relation to each other, until I have a plot that seems to make sense. Or I might start by writing about the headings, linking them back to the practice narrative and elaborating on the experience, or trying to link the headings together through a new narrative. I draft and redraft the account until it comes nearer to the knowledge generated within the emotion of the experience and a possible explanation; 'writing myself to understanding' (Heinrich 1992, p.17).

Step 2 Attend to the feelings – finding what is in your heart

When re-reading the reflective account, I remembered the dread I felt when I walked into Edna's room and how this was provoked by the starkness of the room. I was concerned that this might be signalling that I was going to find that Edna was not being very well cared for. I also remembered the feeling of anxiety that I experienced when Edna's son caught me as I was leaving the ward – in my mind I had moved onto my next visit and was not expecting to speak to her son at that point. I know from previous reflective accounts of my practice that these feelings are part of the process by which I prepare myself for the forthcoming interaction with patients and family members. They are the consequences of me emotionally bracing myself for what will follow (Duke 2007). The dread I felt when

I entered Edna's room braced me for perhaps finding someone that might be receiving suboptimal care. The anxiety I felt when I met Edna's son braced me for the conversation that I was anticipating about what the doctor had said and my duty to protect Edna's confidentiality. However, what is particularly noticeable in this instance is that these emotions are not included in the account (they arise for me through the reading of the account) and moreover, the emotional tone of the account is quite measured, fairly monotone. There are no expressions of passion or distress, no extremes of emotion. This is congruent with the nature of my practice. My practice is intentionally emotionally measured. I suspend my emotional reaction in order to be receptive and sensitive to the emotional nature of people's experience. Elsewhere I describe this as being about: '… being still and receptive to the person's being … recognising and holding their distress, creating safety in which to express feelings' (Duke 2007, p.137).

There is some evidence of the emotional reactions I suspend, and those I allow to be expressed, from the analysis. This evidence occurs in two places.

When I walked into Edna's room I felt dread (remembered and evoked through the reading of the text; an emotional response not reported as experienced in the text). When I left the ward, I felt confident that Edna would soon be comfortable (expressed in the text through my respect for the ward and nursing team).

> *I am deeply impressed*
> *by the doctor's*
> *compassion and clear communication,*
> *by the gentle pace of his conversation,*
> *by the way that he answered questions*
> *and his concern for Edna's family.*
>
> *I am deeply impressed*
> *by the staff nurse's confidence*
> *in the pain management plan*
> *and her speed in putting it into action.*
>
> *… I am planning to come back later*
> *… but I anticipated that [Edna]*
> *would be much more comfortable by then.*

When Edna's son started to talk to me I felt anxious (expressed in the text as concern). When I left the ward I was reassured and impressed by his love and confidence in his mum (remembered on re-reading the text, but not expressed in the text).

> *On the way out of the ward*
> *I am caught by Edna's son.*

I am concerned.
I have not asked Edna...

I am concerned
that it might be too soon to do so...

In contrast...

...He shows his respect for his mum by
explaining that he knows his mum
will let him know
what she wants him to know.

Step 3 Re-evaluate the experience – putting my heart and mind into knowing my practice

For Boud *et al.* (1985), re-evaluation of experience involves making links between previous experiences with those being reflected upon (*association*), making sense of these links – what they contribute to your experiential knowledge (*integration*), testing the links out in some way – for example, through referral to empirical knowledge or by trying out the robustness of the ideas in other reflective accounts (*validation*) and finally making the new emergent knowledge part of your knowledge base – drawing on it in practice, for example (*appropriation*). For me, in following this framework, there is one important difference. Instead of treating the first step (attend to the feelings) as a way of removing feelings that might obstruct a constructive understanding the experience (Boud and Walker 1993), I tend to use them as a starting place in understanding the experience.

Association – making links

The dread I felt when I entered Edna's room was prompted by the starkness of the room. This reminded me (*association*) of the potential power of the physical environment to convey something other than the reality of what is being experienced. In this case, I interpreted the stark room to suggest that Edna was not being well cared for and that her invisibility under the bedclothes suggested a frail older person unable to voice her experience. On the contrary I found the opposite:

Edna curled up in bed,
tiny and barely visible,
hidden under a sheet,
pale nightdress around her neck.

Chapter 7

In contrast...
Edna's face comes alive
and I quickly find
a spirited personality,
a quick intellect
and honed interpersonal skills.

Integration – understanding the importance of links

Furthermore, the account tells me why the physical environment has importance to my expertise (*integration*):

> *There are no clues to help me know Edna,*
> *just this blank, dark and somewhat empty space.*

Edna's room was empty of clues to her identity and to her experience:

> *no cards on the off-white walls*

When I first meet someone, I look for things like cards and photographs because, first of all, I have Chris Johns' words in my ear – 'who is this person?' – the first step in his description of patient assessment (Johns 2000), and because, second, a wise health visitor once taught me to look at the artefacts around a person to come to know that person. She held the view that individuals displayed personal effects such as cards and photographs to ensure that what matters to them is known to others. Often these kinds of clues help me to know how to craft my practice so that it is congruent with the story of who they are as a person. Aranda and Street (1999) express this well in their account of their research with palliative care nurses about what makes practice therapeutic. They describe an important quality in such relationships as attaining a balance between 'being authentic and being a chameleon'. I want to be authentic to my belief (and nursing knowledge) that what matters most is the person, to understand what is of importance to them, to not let the medical story become the only story of importance:

> *We talked about*
> *what was of importance*
> *to her and her family*

In order to do this, I need to shape or colour my practice (be a chameleon) to be congruent with who that person is, so that the person can express this importance. Yet in this instance I had no clue to what kind of approach would be most respectful to Edna's identity before I started to talk to her. Therefore, I needed to take a risk when I initiated the conversation in the approach I took, to hope that a gentle measured start would provoke a response that would enable me to shift my approach to something more closely attuned to her identity. This measured start is demonstrated in the paced way that I describe how I approached Edna:

> *I go around the bed*
> *to the side that Edna is facing*
> *kneel down beside her*
> *take her hand*
> *and introduce myself*

The reflective exemplar demonstrates a mismatch between what I have learnt to use, to come to know a situation, and what is now typically available in acute clinical settings. Hospitals are busy places. Patients frequently move from one bed space to another and from one ward to another, in order to manage the pressure on beds and the clinical needs of those admitted. It is therefore unlikely that people will have personal effects around them expressing who they are and what is of importance to them. This means that a cue which is important to my immediate heuristic understanding of a situation is rarely now available. In other words, some of the (environmental) knowledge on which I have constructed my expertise (my ability to quickly understand a situation) is often missing or may no longer be relevant. However, I continue to interpret their absence as being indicative of a situation where someone may not be receiving good care, whereas they are more likely to be indicative of current clinical environment pressures. I have fallen into what Schön (1983) describes as a 'pattern of error'.

Furthermore, continuing to link a lack of cues to a person's identity and the quality of care they are receiving is detrimental to me as a clinician. Each time it happens, it provokes anxiety and a feeling of dread, because it is important to me that people receive the best and most appropriate care possible. As a consequence, practice becomes increasingly emotionally draining. Furthermore, continuing to practise in this way, trying to manage the mismatch between my clinical experiences and the knowledge which informs my expertise, can result in disengagement in practice, rigidity in thinking and even boredom or burnout (Schön 1983).

What I need to do is to reprogramme my expertise – to de-emphasise or relabel the cues I am picking up and reinterpret them – to cease making a link between a lack of artefacts and a potential lack of care. Paradoxically, it demands time for reflection to achieve this reprogramming. Yet the amount of emotional energy I have to do this work is reduced by the increase in emotional energy needed to manage the anxiety provoked by the kinds of situations I need to reflect upon, to achieve this realignment and an increased workload. Furthermore, it is challenged by belief that, although I appreciate why clinical environments may be devoid of any note of the person being cared for, this void is potentially detrimental to the health of individuals – understandable, but potentially detrimental. Environments influence health (King's Fund 2000).

The account also tells me of the central importance of interrelational practice to expertise. I gained an understanding of Edna's personality and her identity through the conversations that I had with her and her son – *she tells me…*, *we talked about…*. Edna told me about her understanding of why she was in hospital; her understanding of her illness. We talked about what was of most concern to her – her family, being more comfortable, the nature of her pain experience, how she was sleeping, her response to the registrar's news. This enabled me to talk with the medical and nursing team to design an effective pain management plan. Talking with Edna also enabled me to tailor my involvement with the medical and nursing team to one which was concordant with the skills they were demonstrating in her care. It helped me to avoid negating these skills by assuming an expert position. Instead, I was able to adopt a position in which I guided an extension to the decisions they had already instigated, such as those related to Edna's pain management and the psychosocial support they were providing.

Validation – testing out the links

I want to say a couple of things about my understanding of validation before moving onto achieve this phase of Boud *et al.*'s (1985) model of reflection. Validation is not used here in the sense of needing to prove the validity (trust) of something. Rather, I take it to mean to broaden or synthesise understanding, always with the intention of enhancing the range of possible meanings and explanations of practice, and to examine the adequacy of my emerging understanding.

I find that there is a real temptation, in this particular place in reflection, to adopt the processes of evidence-based practice (EBP) to validate reflective analysis. What I mean by this is that I am tempted to ask EBP-oriented questions such as: 'What evidence is there for this finding from my reflective analysis?'. However, questions that are in keeping with Boud *et al.*'s meaning of validation go like: 'Have I sufficiently paid attention to all the possible ways of understanding the practice I am reflecting upon?'; 'Have I been sufficiently open-minded about the alternative ways of understanding practice that are revealed by my analysis?'.

What counts as testing out

Turning to the published research literature to find evidence for the thoughts that originate from my reflection results in answers about what works (or for what there is research evidence about), rather than what else might work or how else I might understand this experience. This is because the method of literature searching described within EBP is concerned with finding the best and most specific answer to a question, whereas the validation process in reflection is designed to find alternative and expansive explanations. If I therefore follow an EBP process, I will limit or curtail my reflective analysis (because the best and most specific answer does not enable me to think about alternative possibilities) and this stifles my ability to make connections between my experience and empirical knowledge.

This is not to criticise the notion of EBP. The original conception of this term as meaning the integration of research with judicious clinical decisions (Sackett et al. 1996) is of foremost importance to patient care. But there is also a perception that EBP is only about the quality of research evidence and applying evidence in practice (see Clegg 2005 and Van Zelm 2006 for more detail). This view has tended to be emphasised with government policy and has resulted in the research endeavour of EBP being emphasised (privileged) over the clinical endeavour (Rolfe 2005) and over the craft of practice (Avis and Freshwater 2006).

This research emphasis is persuasive (of course I want to base my practice on the best evidence), but it is only one part of the story. I also want, and need, to ensure that my knowledge base includes all the ways in which practice can be understood, in order to make the most appropriate choices for how to act when I am in practice. This means I need to draw on other kinds of evidence. I need a rich theory repertoire, in order to predict what might happen if I respond in particular ways, or to guide me in producing the outcomes that I think might be those best in keeping with the needs of someone I am caring for. I need a rich understanding of philosophy and psychology in order to understand being human. I need a rich understanding of the social, in order to understand the social contexts in which I work. I need a rich understanding of education in order to act educationally in whatever practice I am engaged. All of these understandings need to constitute my evidence base.

More worryingly, interpreting EBP as the quality of research evidence and the production of research repositions and reinforces practitioners to be receivers of knowledge, rather than creators of knowledge (Gunter 2004). Thus the generation of knowledge from practice can be seen as 'transgressive' (Fox 2003) – many of the comments from students in the reflective poem in Box 7.1 illustrate this tension. I am tempted to follow the question-setting, literature-searching process because it feels the correct way to do things. In other words, I feel as though I am transgressing or, to use Freshwater's (2000) expression, swimming across a current, if I don't.

I think the trick to managing this cross-current is to keep the themes arising from the reflective analysis foremost – to explore the literature in relation to these key themes in order to expand and elaborate on my understanding, rather than following the EBP process to search the literature for evidence of whether my thoughts are 'right'. To summarise, the latter approach subverts the outcomes of reflective analysis to what *is* known (through empirical research enquiry) rather than what *can* be known (through reflective inquiry).

Box 7.3   References drawn upon to support the relationship between reflection and expertise

---

1. Ericsson, K. and Smith, J. (1991) *Towards a General Theory of Expertise*. Cambridge University Press, Cambridge.
2. Benner, P., Tanner, C. and Chesla, C. (2009) *Expertise in Nursing Practice: Caring, Clinical Judgement and Ethics*, 2nd edn. Springer, New York.
3. Morrison, S.M. and Symes, L. (2011) An integrative review of expert nursing practice. *Journal of Nursing Scholarship*, **43**(2), 163–170.
4. Benner, P. (1984) *From Novice to Expert*. Addison-Wesley, Menlo Park, CA.
5. Rolfe, G. (1998) Beyond expertise: reflective and reflexive nursing practice. In: Johns, C. and Freshwater, D. (eds) *Transforming Nursing through Reflective Practice*. Blackwell Science, Oxford, pp.21–31.

What can be known about expertise from my encounter with Edna?

I identified several themes from the reflective analysis to develop my understanding of the relationship between reflection and expertise – the focus of this chapter (*validation*). Here I demonstrate how I have ordered the themes from the reflective analysis and how I have reasoned the salience of these themes in relation to selected literature on expertise. I have not discussed the literature on expertise in any depth because although my reading of these sources has framed this reasoning, my purpose here is to illustrate the process of validation rather than the outcome – the references for these sources are provided in Box 7.3 should you wish to follow these up. What is also important to remember is that this is not an inclusive overview of what has been written about expertise (and neither should it be), because it focuses upon the themes arising from the selected practice example. Other practice examples will illustrate other themes about expertise.

Theme 1

The meaning of the environmental cues to patient care, on which I have built my expertise, require re-examination and 'reprogramming'. Therefore:

- expertise is a continual process of refinement and adaptation[1]
- expertise is never absolute – it is not a state or something that is attained, like a role, but something that is expressed and refined through practice.[2]

Theme 2

The meaning of the environmental cues on which I have built my expertise were, at one time in my clinical life, relevant. However, they are not currently relevant to the clinical context in which I practise. Therefore:

- expertise is situational and temporal – it is developed at particular moments of time, through particular circumstances and contexts and is therefore applicable to similar moments and contexts[2]
- expertise may not always be transferable to other moments in time and other contexts.

Theme 3

However, although the clinical context has changed, the process of my practice still seems to be congruent with the nature of practice – there is nothing different in this reflective account to the uncertainty that I have experienced in other accounts and the conversational process of practice I analysed in other accounts. Therefore I believe:

- expertise is about working with uncertainty – the uncertainty of what I will find when I go to meet someone and in how they, their family, and healthcare practitioners will respond[3]
- expertise depends on interrelational practice, and the skill to craft a conversation that is respectful to others, of their knowledge and being, and yet contributes to what might be helpful to the knowledge I need to provide care and to so do with authenticity.[3]

Theme 4

The reflective processes described above have enabled me to expand my understanding of my expertise and the knowledge by which it is informed. Therefore:

- expertise can be known – it is not just unconscious knowing of practice.[4] The unconscious knowledge can be brought to the surface and become reknown, recrafted, and known to others[5]
- the reflective processes by which expertise can be known have logic.[5] They are rational in the sense that they are methodical, providing a method of reasoning that enables possibilities for understanding practice
- reflection and expertise are intrinsically and intentionally entwined in clinical scholarship.[3]

Chapter 7

Appropriation – embracing my learning from my encounter with Edna

Appropriation, the final process in re-evaluating the experience, is about making the practice knowledge, identified from the reflective analysis, my own – embracing it and letting it influence the position I occupy in relation to reflective practice and expertise. This is a bit scary because embracing this practice knowledge means acknowledging that there are some dents in my expertise, places where it would be wise to be cautious in practice. In addition, the means of repairing these dents relies on both sufficient clinical experiences to test out new ways of understanding the clinical environment, but also sufficient time and emotional energy to engage in critical reflection to guide this process, neither of which are easy to come by.

There is no reflection yet to share on how I am getting on with this – as I write, I am waiting for my clinical contract to be renewed, so it has not been possible to test what the necessary change feels like or to see whether I can be aware of the prompts in practice that I have discussed as they appear and retune my thinking. But it is my plan to have a go as soon as I am able.

Nevertheless, there are some things (other kinds of association) that I have learnt and relearnt about reflection as a consequence of writing this chapter, which I wish to comment upon. I said at the beginning of the chapter that I am finding being reflective a big 'ask', but that I thought that the only way I could reflect the difficulty of this 'ask' was by trusting the process of reflection. This means that I have needed to be embedded in the reflective process, head deep underneath the cross-current that Freshwater (2000) describes, allowing myself to feel the pull of the competing currents, to sometimes feel swamped by the emotional weight of these currents and the fear that I might not get to the surface, or find a way through to the meaning of the experience I was analysing, and to the end of the chapter. Overall, I have felt continually emotionally drained by this experience, by the emotional effort of writing an authentic account of practice, the effort of carefully analysing the account and considering the resulting knowledge.

In addition, and perhaps as a consequence of this emotional weight, I frequently came to places where I felt a hiatus, a block to knowing where to go next. Sometimes this was because I had run out of emotional energy, given that this writing was being juggled with the pressures of a busy work and family life, and by professional and personal bereavements. Consequently, when I sat down to write, I often found that I could not find my reflective spirit. At these times I have needed to wait until I had the emotional space to continue. Other times it was because I was paralysed by the feeling of being an imposter that I discussed in the introduction. At these times I have needed to remind myself to trust the process of reflection, and to respect what I could learn by careful analysis and by being open to this opportunity.

Thus this reflective experience adds to my knowledge about the personal cost of reflection that I have discussed in previous editions of this book, and the need to respect personal ebbs and flows in order to work with the emotion of reflection (Duke and Copp 1994; Duke 2004). Reflection is not easy, particularly in the current clinical context. It needs support, emotional energy and self-awareness. As Boud and Walker (1993) note, the absence of these things readily blocks reflection.

The experience of feeling the weight of reflection, and the difficulty of being reflective, is in complete contrast to what I have gained from being reflective and to my enthusiasm and support for reflective practice. Already, my sense of expertise is more in balance as a consequence of this reflective analysis. I know that as I accommodate this understanding within my self-concept of being a nurse and as having expertise, the scales will tip more towards the joy of reflection and of being a nurse than the emotional weight of these experiences.

Concluding reflections

Reflection has been a companion in my quest for expertise for a long time now. This journey has embraced the knowledge transmitted by reflective accounts and understanding their potential power to silence analysis, the excitement of actively being engaged in learning about my practice, and in finding ways to analyse my practice. This chapter brings me back full circle to the emotional difficulty of reflection and the courage required to act on the consequences.

Nevertheless, I cannot imagine being a nurse without drawing on the process of reflection. As Boykin (1998, p.45) argues, reflective practice is essential 'to truly nurse'. I believe too that it is also essential to truly educate. Reflection is the means through which I assess what is 'right', how I assess the moral quality of my practice and the stance I take as a practitioner within both my clinical and educational practice. For example, in my experience of caring for Edna I was concerned with the quality of her care, for the environment in which she was cared for; I judged the compassion she was shown by the ward and medical team, and the respect demonstrated by her son. I was, in short, concerned with whether we were getting things 'right' for her. This moral assessment is about rights, equity, freedom and justice (Carr and Kemmis 1986; Mezirow 1991). It involves understanding of how the social context influences practice and how practice is known (Carr and Kemmis 1986). It demands that I understand the contextual influences on care, and on education, and have the ability and courage to challenge and change these influences for the better.

However, what this reflective analysis has shown is that it is difficult to be reflective when you are caught in the in-between (Ferrell 1998), whether this is the space between patient care and the resources needed to provide this care, or the space between the need to reflect and the emotional energy to do so, or the space between clinical practice wisdom and the knowledge generated by research or the space between different organisations. Nevertheless, whilst such in-between spaces might threaten my ability to enact my morality, this is not a sufficient reason not to reflect. As Taylor (1975) states in his exploration of the principles of ethics:

> 'A moral agent may not always fulfil the requirements of a moral standard or rule; that is he need not be morally perfect. But he must have the capacity to judge himself on the basis of such a criterion and to use it as a guide to his choice and conduct'. (p.6)

Thus reflection is also the means by which I know that something is not right; to use the skills of reflection to assess the status quo and to find the constraining factors within it (Taylor 1998, p.134). It seems to me that in the current context of healthcare, the current crush on nursing resources constrains and potentially oppresses the potential for reflection by squeezing out any energy that might be used for this purpose. Our potential to influence care is subsequently threatened. It therefore requires us to be even more determined to be reflective, so that nursing voices influence care, as a consequence of knowing how to care, rather than allowing this voice to be oppressed. It requires me as an educator to equip the nurses with whom I work with well-honed reflective skills in reflection and to walk the talk, to walk alongside them in their reflective journeys, to help them to galvanise the courage they need to challenge practice and to model how to raise this challenge. It requires me to challenge how reflection is interpreted within the University, to model how clinical and empirical knowledge can be integrated, and to inspire and stand with my academic colleagues in the journey to embrace this fuller understanding of reflection. A big 'ask' indeed, but one that we need to embrace as strongly, and as surely, as we did when we started on the journey of writing about reflection, in those heady times, all those years ago.

References

Aitchinson, J. and Graham, P. (1989) Potato crisp pedagogy. In: Cristicos, C. (ed) *Experiential Learning in Formal and Non-formal Learning*. University of Natal Media Resource Centre, Durban, pp.15–21.

Aranda, S. and Street, A.F. (1999) On being authentic and being a chameleon: nurse–patient interactions revisited. *Nursing Inquiry*, **6**(2), 75–82.

Avis, M. and Freshwater, D. (2006) Evidence for practice, epistemology and critical reflection. *Nursing Philosophy*, **7**, 216–224.

Boykin, A. (1998) Nursing as caring through the reflective lens. In: Johns, C. and Freshwater, D. (eds) *Transforming Nursing Through Reflective Practice*. Blackwell Science, Oxford, pp.43–50.

Chapter 7

Boud, D. and Walker, D. (1993) Barriers to reflection on experience. In: Boud, D., Cohen, R. and Walker, D. (eds) *Using Experience for Learning*. Open University Press, Buckingham, pp.73–86.

Boud, D., Keogh, R. and Walker, D. (1985) Promoting reflection in learning: a model. In Boud, D., Keogh, R. and Walker, D. (eds) *Reflection: Turning Experience into Learning*. Kogan Page, London, pp.18–40.

Boyd, E.M. and Fales, A.W. (1983) Reflecting learning: key to learning from experience. *Journal of Humanistic Psychology*, **23**(2), 99–117.

Carr, J.M. (2003) Poetic expressions of vigilance. *Qualitative Health Research*, **13**(9), 1324–1331.

Carr, W. and Kemmis, S. (1986) *Becoming Critical*. Falmer Press, London.

Clegg, S. (2005) Evidence-based practice in educational research: a critical realist critique of systematic review. *British Journal of Sociology of Education*, **26**(3), pp.415–428.

Crepeau, E. (2000) Reconstructing Gloria: a narrative analysis of team meeting. *Qualitative Health Research*, **10**(6), 766–787.

Cristicos, C. (1993) Experiential learning and social transformation for a post-apartheid learning future. In: Boud, D., Cohen, R. and Walker, D. (eds) *Using Experience for Learning*. Open University Press, Buckingham, pp.157–168.

Duke, S. (2000) The experience of becoming reflective. In: Burns, S. and Bulman, C. (eds) *Reflective Practice in Nursing*, 2nd edn. Blackwell Science, Oxford, pp.137–155.

Duke, S. (2004) When reflection becomes a cul-de-sac: strategies for finding the focus and moving on. In: Bulman, C. and Schutz, S. (eds) *Reflective Practice in Nursing*, 3rd edn. Wiley-Blackwell, Oxford, pp.146–160.

Duke, S. (2007) A narrative case study evaluation of the role of nurse consultant in palliative care. PhD thesis, School of Education, University of Southampton.

Duke, S. (2008) Continuing the journey with reflection. In: In: Bulman, C. and Schutz, S. (eds) *Reflective Practice in Nursing*, 4th edn. Wiley-Blackwell, Oxford, pp.189–218.

Duke, S. and Appleton, J.M. (2000) The use of reflection in a palliative care programme: a quantitative study of the development of reflective skills over an academic year. *Journal of Advanced Nursing*, **32**(6), pp.1557–1168.

Duke, S. and Copp, G. (1994) The personal side of reflection. In: Palmer, A., Burns, S. and Bulman, C. (eds) *Reflective Practice: The Growth of the Reflective Practitioner*. Blackwell, Oxford, pp.100–109.

Ferrell, L. (1998) Doing the right thing: customary versus reflective morality. In: Johns, C. and Freshwater, D. (eds) *Transforming Nursing Through Reflective Practice*. Blackwell Science, Oxford, pp.32–42.

Fook, J. and Gardner, F. (2007) *Practising Critical Reflection*. Open University Press, Buckingham.

Fox, N.J. (2003) Practice-based evidence: towards collaborative and transgressive research. *Sociology*, **37**(1), 81–102.

Freshwater, D. (2000) Crosscurrents: against cultural narration in nursing. *Journal of Advanced Nursing*, **32**(3), 695–703.

Glesne, C. (1997) That rare feeling: re-presenting research through poetic transcription. *Qualitative Inquiry*, **3**, 202–221.

Gunter, H. (2004) Labels and labelling in the field of educational leadership. *Discourse: Studies in the Cultural Politics of Education*, **25**(1), 21–41.

Heinrich, K.T. (1992) The intimate dialogue: journal writing by students. *Nurse Educator*, **17**(6), 17–21.

Johns, C. (2000) *Becoming a Reflective Practitioner*. Blackwell, Oxford.

King's Fund (2000) *Enhancing the Healing Environment*. King's Fund, London.

Mezirow, J. (1991) *Fostering Critical Reflection in Adulthood*. Jossey-Bass, San Francisco.

Richardson, L. (2000) Writing: a method of inquiry. In: Denzin, N. and Lincoln, Y. (eds) *The Handbook of Qualitative Research*. Sage, London, pp.923–948.

Rolfe, G. (2005) The deconstructing angel: nursing, reflection and evidence-based practice. *Nursing Inquiry*, **12**(2), 78–86.

Sackett, D.L., Rosenberg, W., Gray, J., Haynes, R. and Richardson, W. (1996) Evidence-based medicine: what it is and what it is not. *British Medical Journal*, **312**, 71–72.

Schön, D. (1983) *The Reflective Practitioner*. Temple Smith, London.

Taylor, B. (1998) Locating a phenomenological perspective of reflective nursing and midwifery practice by contrasting interpretive and critical reflection. In: Johns, C. and Freshwater, D. (eds) *Transforming Nursing Through Reflective Practice*. Blackwell Science, Oxford, pp.134–150.

Taylor, P.W. (1975) *Principles of Ethics: An Introduction*. Wadsworth, Belmont, CA.

Van Zelm, R. (2006) The bankruptcy of evidence based practice. *International Journal of Evidence-Based Healthcare*, **4**(3), 1.

Chapter 8

Assessing and evaluating reflection

Sue Schutz

Faculty of Health and Life Sciences, Oxford Brookes University, Oxford; University of Southampton, Southampton, UK

Introduction

In this chapter I want to turn your attention to the more structured aspects of reflection – the role of assessment and of evaluation. Reflection, as part of academic or professional courses, is often used as a learning and teaching strategy and as a key professional skill. As an informal activity, outside the classroom, reflection may also be used to facilitate development of new skills in practice. In both situations, assessment could be said to be valuable in order to identify our achievements. Additionally, reflection may be a means to an end or an end in itself but in both cases, some evaluation of the success of the venture is needed. This chapter is written for two groups of readers: those who are starting out with, or engaged in, reflection and need to consider the role of assessment and evaluation of reflection for their own needs, and also for those who facilitate or mentor/coach reflection in an informal or academic setting and need to make assessments of students' abilities.

Sumison and Fleet (1996) stated that little is known about how reflection and reflective practice are best promoted or measured. The body of evidence on reflection has continued to grow since the last edition of this book; however, the assessment and evaluation of reflection remains a contentious area. The aims of this chapter are to define the meanings of assessment and evaluation of reflection in nursing and explore the practical and theoretical issues that this raises. I will also outline and debate the existing evidence base for the assessment and evaluation of reflection.

The lack of clarity about the process of assessing reflection can be seen as an obstacle in its promotion (Newell 1994) and this poses difficulties for those of us to whom assessment and evaluation of reflection is a necessity. The current emphasis in healthcare on evidence-based practice

Reflective Practice in Nursing, Fifth Edition. Edited by Chris Bulman and Sue Schutz.
© 2013 John Wiley & Sons, Ltd. Published 2013 by John Wiley & Sons, Ltd.

makes this lack of evidence a pertinent issue and many authors raise this (e.g. Mallik 1998; Paget 2001). Evidence, standards and targets are a constant pressure on health and social care professionals and can often be perceived as being counterforces to reflective practice. However, some educationalists suggest the need to *marry* organisational goals with goals for reflection (Valli 1993; Korthagen and Wubbels 1995), so the two are not necessarily mutually exclusive. Definitions of reflection will inevitably differ depending on the social factors influencing the development of organisations and collaborating practice areas, but reflective and organisational goals can complement each other; after all, the aims are the same.

Definitions

Discussion about definitions of assessment and evaluation of reflection may begin with the debate about what reflection actually is. Chapter 1 highlights the requirement to gain an appreciation of what reflection means and offers an explanation of the concept, drawing on a number of useful sources. The key thing is to pay attention to how the meaning of reflection is identified within nursing and thus develop more of an appreciation of the similarities and differences in interpretations. This means doing a lot more sharing between institutions on how we are tackling assessment and evaluation of reflection and, of course, it means doing more research.

In addition, Chapter 2 on reflective skills presents some putative attributes of reflective practice that may help educators to make more sound assessments. Moreover, you may like to have a look at the work of Korthagen and Wubbels (1995) who reported on a programme of research exploring the mathematics department of a teacher education college in The Netherlands, where the fundamental goal of the programme was the promotion of reflective teaching. They define reflection from the cognitive perspective as a mental process for the structuring or restructuring of an experience, problem or existing knowledge and insights. They indicate the importance of relating this to views about good teaching, which they capture through their research as having a good command of the subject but also the importance of nurturing good interpersonal relationships with students and an awareness of one's own functioning as a teacher. Thus facilitation, focusing on real and concrete problems, problem solving and learning how to learn were all key values in the programme teachers' views of good teaching. Their acknowledgement of the need to consider the link between concepts of reflective practice and good teaching is a valuable pointer in exploring the development of reflective practice in nursing, since I would suggest that practitioners' understandings of reflection will undoubtedly arise from their beliefs about good nursing.

From the summary of their research, these authors suggest a series of critical attributes and correlates of reflection based on their explicit views of good teaching and reflection.

Attributes

- A reflective teacher is capable of structuring situations and problems and considers it important to do so.
- A reflective teacher uses certain standard questions when structuring experiences such as: What happened? Why did it happen? What did I do wrong? What could I have done differently?
- A reflective teacher can easily answer the question of what he or she wants to learn. S/he is less dependent on educators when it comes to choosing learning goals.
- A reflective teacher can adequately describe and analyse his or her own functioning in interpersonal relationships with others.

Correlates

- Reflective teachers have better interpersonal relationships with students than other teachers.
- Reflective teachers develop a high degree of job satisfaction.
- Reflective teachers also consider it important for their students to learn by investigating and structuring things themselves.
- Reflective teachers have previously been encouraged to structure their experiences and problems.
- Reflective teachers have strong feelings of personal security and self-efficacy.
- Teachers with teaching experience, who have a high degree of self-efficacy, focus in their reflections about their teaching on their students. When they have a low sense of self-efficacy, they focus on themselves.
- Reflective teachers appear to talk or write relatively easily about their experiences.

If you are a teacher or facilitator of reflection, I think you will find this very illuminating. It has a high degree of credibility for both teachers and practitioners. If as facilitators of reflection, we are to be successful, it is important that we 'walk the walk' as well as 'talking the talk'.

At this stage it is important to be clear about the terminology that we are using. The terms 'assessment' and 'evaluation' are sometimes used interchangeably but in the context in which I am going to explore these activities, to continue to use them in this way would be confusing. Burnard (1988) distinguishes between the two in the context of reflective journal writing. He states that to assess is to: 'identify a particular state at a particular time, usually with a view to taking action to change or modify that state' (p.105) and that evaluation is to: 'place a value on a course of action, to identify the success or otherwise of a course of action' (p.105).

With this in mind, we can see that to assess reflection and to evaluate are two rather different activities. Indeed, they have different aims, processes and structures. The assessment of reflection may involve a different group of people from those involved in evaluation, and the timing is likely to differ too. Commonly, when the assessment of reflection is raised, this refers to the ways in which students undertaking educational activities are tested in their ability to reflect on their own and others' practice. It embraces the process of reflection, the possession of the skills for reflection and the outcomes of reflection in terms of practice change. An example of this would be the assessment of a student's written reflection on her own practice in a portfolio. The assessor uses specific tools in order to make a judgement about the level of reflection achieved.

In talking about the evaluation of reflection, I will be referring to activities that aim to uncover the *value of reflection* in the educational curriculum or in nursing practice. An example of this might be the annual review of a nursing degree programme by the higher education organisation, which asks the programme team to undertake a review of the use of reflection in that course or an evaluation of the use of reflective groups in the practice area.

The assessment of reflection

Many aspects of nursing practice and education have an impact on the assessment of reflection, in particular, the settings in which students are currently engaged in practice. This may be within an institution or in the community, but it is always within the broad framework of health and social care. The complexities of the health service are familiar to us all, but it is worth spending some time exploring what it is about a health or social care setting that has an impact on reflective practice and assessment.

The healthcare context

This encompasses the healthcare organisation as a whole and the quality of leadership and management within that organisation. Constant change within health and social care is a fact of life and it is generally recognised that this perpetual motion is due to the impact of political, technological and sociological drivers. In nursing, the situational or contextual setting of practice is of paramount importance and reflection can play a key part in helping the student to connect with the realities of practice. Students need to be equipped with the necessary skills that will help them learn from what they see and experience; the influence of the context can be very powerful. Staff in practice who are supervising students in reflective practice are also affected by these changes. The availability of quality, motivated mentors for students may be compromised, despite service/ education agreements and learning opportunities thus impinged upon.

At many universities, factors such as these have contributed to the continual review and development of programmes to prepare nurses and other healthcare professionals for first level and advanced practice. In particular, it has led to the development of changes in relation to the assessment of reflection through academic work and the use of innovative tools such as portfolios to map student development. Additionally, increased interest in the dialogic approach to reflection has meant that higher education institutes have introduced reflective assessment.

Issues in assessing reflection

The great debate in the literature is about whether reflection should be assessed at all or whether it is a contradiction in terms to make judgements about what is a rather personal process. This goes to the heart of the role that reflection plays in the development of the skills needed for practice. If reflection is a key skill in achieving the learning outcomes of particular courses and is acknowledged to have a positive impact on care, then I believe it must be assessed. The literature describes the assessment of reflection in both summative (for example, Morgan and Johns 2005) and formative (Getliffe 1996) ways and indicates the tensions that are about both assessment of reflection *per se* and about the tools.

Rich and Parker (1995) discussed the potential for what they call *psychological burn* when adding assessment to the (possibly painful) process of reflection. This suggests that there may be actual or potential harm in attempting to make judgements about students' abilities to reflect and adds an imperative to the debate about whether it should be done at all, and if it is, how to do it 'safely'. Indeed, Cotton (2001) goes further in likening reflection to the confessional, where someone else knows one's innermost thoughts and where one may be judged.

These are concerns to be taken seriously but the fact remains that nurses (and other professionals) value professional knowledge through reflection because they recognise the problem of the theory–practice gap and are struggling to do something about it. If nurse education does not work at ways to assess and evaluate reflection successfully, propositional knowledge will continue to dominate as the only legitimate form of knowledge in higher education. The value of informal or culturally specific knowledge can be enhanced and made legitimate through its use in practice (Eraut 1994) and through reflection.

There is a dilemma here in what is wanted for the purposes of assessment; is it the spontaneous, immediate response to a practice event or is it the considered reaction of later? Both are reflective. What needs to be considered is the emotional element of reflection. If time could be thought to remove or alter this, then timely reflection is most important, as emotions are a valid aspect of reflection. Some students find it useful to go back to a diary and use the benefit of hindsight to edit their reflection for the purposes of assessment. Thus they may not be writing spontaneously when being assessed, but they are able to make use of verbal, more immediate reflection with colleagues and mentors at the time and then write at a later date.

The work undertaken by Ashford *et al.* (1998) found that students were freer to take risks in reflection when no formal assessment is taking place. This would suggest that a more meaningful level of reflection might be possible where no judgement is going to be made. However, when reflection is used formally in courses to develop practice, some type of assessment needs to be made in order to best utilise and map that progress; it is difficult to see how this can be avoided. This is where the use of both formative as well as summative strategies can be helpful. Chapter 3 by Sylvina Tate discusses the use of reflective journals and highlights the fact that not all of what is written in a reflective journal or diary may be used for formal assessment purposes. Therefore, the structure of the assessment of reflection needs to be formulated in such a way that there is opportunity for students to have both a private and a public 'version' of their reflective thoughts.

However, it should not be assumed that the assessment of reflection in students is a kind of 'necessary evil'; Paget (2001) found that the impact of reflection on practice seemed to be enhanced by summative assessment, possibly because it is a motivator to effective reflection. Yet, it could just be a motivator for students to get something written even if it is of little value, so we need to be careful about putting too much pressure on students to come up with a product. Another key question that arises here is the clarity about what is actually being assessed. Both Goodman (1984) and Mezirow (1991) assert that there are levels of reflection and therefore, without formal assessment, the level (or depth) to which an individual student is able to reflect on practice cannot be known.

It is important that educators and practitioners are clear about the outcomes of the effort put into reflection by students. Clearly, it is a time-consuming activity and one that carries with it an element of risk to those involved. Ghaye and Lillyman (2010) have asserted that reflection must have a tangible outcome and this is difficult to measure without some form of assessment. This brings me to the second issue, which is how reflection might be best assessed. I noted earlier that the notion of 'private' and 'public' versions of reflective writing might be a possible answer; Hannigan (2001) sees assessment of reflection as one part of a comprehensive assessment strategy and that how it is done is key. Hannigan also advocates attention to the preparation of assessors and to the support of students and staff during the process.

In summary, where reflection is a key part of the curriculum, it needs to be assessed formally. However, the strategy used to achieve this must include both summative and formative elements, and be framed by a support system for students and assessors.

Problems with the assessment of reflection

The problem areas associated with assessing reflection are many and varied, as might be expected. The wide interpretations of what constitutes reflection and how it is practically applied make for a minefield of difficulties. The key challenges that might arise are listed below.

- Clarification of what the organisation understands by reflection
- A decision about whether it is the process of reflection or its outcome that should be assessed
- Consideration of whether reflection has levels and how these develop over time
- Addressing the barriers to honesty caused by assessment
- A lack of effective tools for assessment
- The skills of available facilitators
- The relative political and financial pressures

I will briefly consider each of these problem areas in turn.

Clarifying what we mean by reflection

The varied interpretations of what constitutes good reflection are a problem in that students need to know what is expected of them and assessors need to know what they are looking for. However, there is an overlap in terms such as reflection, reflective practice, reflective learning, critical thinking and critical analysis (Daly 1998). Some of these are used interchangeably and some are aspects of others. Many of the skills needed for reflection, such as self-awareness and analysis, are required by more than one of these concepts. Some of the expected outcomes are also common – the improvement of practice and professional development, for example. What is important is that educational teams have a clear idea of what they mean by reflection, that this is based on the best available evidence and that this is passed on to students using it. The putative attributes of reflective practice, outlined in Chapter 2, may be of some assistance but it is probably best not to confuse reflection and reflective practice at this point.

Assessing the process or the outcome of reflection

Burton (2000) asks whether written reflective accounts accurately demonstrate learning and development or are merely 'a perfunctory exercise to comply with … requirements' (p.105). Here, she raises the question of what is actually being assessed: the process of reflecting on practice or the impact that this reflection has on the individual's practice. There is no doubt that those students who possess good academic writing skills are at an advantage when written reflection is being assessed and there is a danger that students write what they think the assessor wants to hear

(Platzer *et al.* 2000a,b). This echoes Hannigan's (2001) call for comprehensive assessment strategies, which can take account of these challenges by adopting a variety of testing strategies. What is desirable is for students to engage fruitfully in reflective practice – not for them to jump through hoops. Therefore, it is both the process and the outcome that are being assessed because they are both of equal importance.

Developing reflecting levels

When assessing students' acquisition of reflective skills, we need to take into account the speed at which students develop these skills over time. Reflection is a complex activity and those new to reflection may have difficulty with it. Indeed, it is clear that some are more naturally reflective than others and many students struggle with reflective practice for a long time. Glaze (2002) found that, in the early stages of learning to reflect, a lack of insight acted as a barrier to reflective development, and assessment during these early stages needs to take this into account. In postgraduate courses and for mature students, this is often not the case because these students are usually more experienced and confident people, so individual evaluation of where the students 'start at' may be needed. Burrows (1995) suggested that those under 25 years of age might lack the cognitive readiness and experience for reflective practice. This is likely to include many undergraduate nursing students. However, Burrows focuses on cognition, whereas reflection is the intermingling of thinking, feeling and action so perhaps other studies focusing more on this mix may reveal a different perspective. What is important is that an assessor looks for a rounded sense of the student's reflective ability, not simply a sum of the criteria used to assess it.

Barriers to honesty

Reflection is a highly personal exercise and it is clear that bringing personal feelings and judgements into the public domain may act as a barrier to reflection. Bolton (2010) maintains that assessment undermines effective reflection and that honesty will be compromised by any attempts to bring it into public view. In my experience, this can often be a problem but other forms of reflection may provide the student with an opportunity to reflect more openly and we can find ways of including these alternatives in assessed work without the student feeling exposed. The use of individual tutorials, reflective groups, action learning circles and personal diaries can all give students the chance to 'try it out' in a safe environment and, hopefully, come to terms with a level of honesty that feels comfortable and aids effective reflection. Mentors and clinical supervisors also have a key role to play in encouraging honest and open reflection in their students; this is, of course, dependent on a positive relationship where trust and communication are fostered.

The perceived lack of effective tools for assessment

The range of tools available for the assessment of reflection includes journals, learning contracts, critical incident analyses and reflective essays. For formative assessment, action learning circles, group and individual tutorials may be used. One of the problems that can arise with these methods is a lack of clarity about what is being assessed. It is important to have criteria that reflect the skills and activities necessary for effective reflection and to build in room for development over time. On postgraduate programmes, where educators are working with more experienced practitioners, problems can still arise. As Hannigan (2001) pointed out, these people are often experts in their area and use an embedded or tacit form of knowledge and thus can find it difficult to articulate what they do. Reflection can be, and often is, found by these students to be a way of articulating and making concrete this informal knowledge. Additionally, attending seminars on reflection does not necessarily equip practitioners to do it (Paget 2001); participation in the process is what is important.

Tools designed to assess reflection need to be flexible enough to allow students to progress at their own speed and to demonstrate their abilities to reflect in a variety of ways. Burton (2000) points out that coercion may defeat the purpose of the exercise and lead to demotivation so we need to use a variety of tools and allow for various speeds of progression. Anxiety and poor memory (Reece-Jones 1995; Andrews et al. 1998) can also adversely affect performance and the tools used to assess reflection need to allow students to perform to the best of their ability despite these barriers.

Skills of facilitators

The role of the reflective learning facilitator is crucial and can make or break a reflective experience. This may be a lecturer, link lecturer, lecturer practitioner, practice teacher, mentor, supervisor, colleague or manager; they all require very specific skills. A facilitator might not also be the assessor and in fact, this may be a good thing because it can 'muddy the waters' if they are. However, mentors who are assessing students using reflective methods such as guided reflection in practice are often in a position of both facilitating and assessing, just as lecturers often are. The problems inherent in this situation include a lack of understanding or familiarity with reflection and with the assessment process (McCarthy and Murphy 2008). A programme of training and ongoing development for those who assess reflection is important and this needs to be well resourced. Facilitators need to have some experience of reflection and be able to offer students a balance of support and challenge. They also need to have expertise in the student's field of practice so that they can understand the contextual issues that influence student experiences. Research tells us that training of facilitators and their own experiences of using reflection are crucial to the success of assessing reflection in students (Duffy 2008).

Some helpful material related specifically to facilitating assessing reflection may be found in Andrews *et al.* (1998) and Durgahee (1998). The role of the facilitator in balancing the dual imperatives of facilitating and assessing may be aided by a stronger focus on formative assessment rather than the more traditional summative or final assessment. Facilitators reading this chapter will find help in other parts of this book, particularly Chapters 4, 5, 6 and 9.

Political and financial pressures

The never-ending financial and resource pressures placed upon nurses can often be seen to impact negatively on our ability to effectively assess reflection in students and others. It is without doubt a time-consuming activity that can be relegated in a busy care environment to last on the list of priorities. This can be due to many factors, some of which are not directly related to real pressures. Fears in clinical staff about facilitating reflection can result in excuses about time pressures and educators need to be sure that those asked to facilitate are adequately prepared and supported. Anxiety is created through the conflicting needs of patient care, students' expectations and the demands of managers and administrators.

In the absence of a clear evidence base for reflective practice, it is often not afforded the necessary time. More research is needed which could indicate the potential benefits of reflection for patient care, and for service delivery in general. However, it would be hard to disagree with the notion of equipping nurses with critical thinking skills. Equipping them with reflective skills simply takes this a few steps further since not only are we supporting and challenging students to develop their critical thinking, we are also concerned with facilitating them to develop their critical self-awareness and motivation to positively challenge and change practice, ultimately for the benefit of clients.

Tools for assessing reflection

A number of tools are available to assess students' reflective abilities and it is likely that an educational curriculum will utilise a range of these, as each has strengths in the assessment of aspects of reflection. Many of these are also suitable for use in an informal setting, where reflection may be assessed as part of professional development, perhaps for clinical supervision or appraisal purposes too. The variety of tools can be divided into verbal and written strategies.

Verbal strategies:

- reflective discussion with mentors
- individual and group reflective tutorials
- action learning circles

Written strategies:

- reflective learning contract
- critical incident analysis
- reflective essay
- reflective journal or diary
- reflective case study
- the reflective portfolio

Each of these has its own distinct process and form; I will say a few words about each in turn, evaluating particular strengths and problem areas. Each will use the terms that are appropriate to reflection in an institute of higher education, but can be appropriate for informal assessment of reflection too, if you are using reflection as part of clinical supervision, for example. For those of you who are starting out or are in engaged in reflection, you will find that the guidance given here and the points raised will give you some help in going about reflection when assessment is part of the journey.

Verbal strategies

Reflective discussion with mentors

The use of reflective dialogue to aid reflection has been the subject of research (see Phillips *et al*. 2000; Van Horn and Freed 2008) and can be planned and structured or spontaneous and timely to the event. Reflective discussion between mentors and students often falls into the unplanned category and is usually related to care, taking place in the context of an event. I have mentioned the advantages of the former but not the impact of reflection in the setting of care. The influence of this is unknown but one would suspect that it might help or hinder the openness of the discussion, dependent upon the particular situation. Mentors may need to be sensitive to this and the spontaneity of the discussion may be affected by the need to find a comfortable and safe place to reflect. These kinds of reflective encounters may not be directly assessed, but they frequently feed into the assessment process. One of the mentor's responsibilities is often to validate competence in certain areas and this is likely to include reflective discussion of related events.

The student will also be developing their thinking and self-awareness in the context of real-life practice and thus reflective discussion in the care setting is likely to be used in the development of assessed written work. The preparation of mentors is key to the success of this strategy and an exploration of reflection should feature in their education. I find that the frameworks of Johns (Johns and Freshwater 2009) and Gibbs (Gibbs *et al*. 1988) are often used (see Chapter 9 for details on these) and may be familiar to mentors. Mentors work alongside students on a day-to-day basis and are familiar with the experiences that they are exposed to. Factors such as workload, the skills of the mentor and the culture and characteristics of the care setting will influence both the frequency of these discussions and their quality. Their success depends heavily on the mentor's confidence in making explicit his/her own thought processes and openness to challenge and debate. Work carried out by Schutz et al. (1996) showed how students perceive the relative success of a placement to depend heavily on the quality of their relationship with the mentor, and thus such qualities directly influence the level of reflective discussion. In Chapter 5, Pam Sharp and Charlotte Maddison discuss many of these points in more detail.

Individual and group tutorials

Individual and group tutorials are a regular feature of programmes for nurse preparation. Yet as resources become stretched, there has been pressure in many universities to minimise one-to-one tutorials, in favour of group work. The reflective tutorial can be used to focus on specific events in a student's life or to address more general issues in practice. Very often, a skilled facilitator can achieve both. The individual tutorial may be used to discuss areas that are problematic to a certain student and therefore not appropriate for groups, whilst group tutorials allow students to participate at the level at which they feel comfortable and to learn from each other. Facilitators of group tutorials need to ensure that students who are reluctant to contribute are not neglected and are able to engage as much as possible with other reflective activities in which they feel more comfortable. A good knowledge of group dynamics and well-developed skills in facilitation are very important; students need to be in a safe and comfortable environment whilst subjects that may be challenging are debated. Heath (1998) suggested that mixing students who are at different stages of a course (and therefore likely to be at different levels of reflective ability) together in a group is of benefit.

The role of reflective tutorials in the assessment of reflection is likely to be of a formative nature, allowing students to explore and develop ideas and to gain feedback on these. Research has been reported on reflective practice groups (see the work reported by Platzer et al. 2001a and b) and this has shown that reflective groups have particular influence on students' development. In Chapter 4, the pros and cons of group reflection are debated in more depth. In many universities, teaching staff have introduced a reflective tutorial group into the curriculum, whereby students meet regularly in the group throughout the period of an undergraduate pre-registration programme. The skills needed for reflection are introduced gradually, starting with the skills of self-awareness and moving through those of description, critical analysis and evaluation. This staged approach is mindful of the concerns expressed by Heath (1998) about how novices can be overwhelmed by the new experience to which they are exposed.

Written strategies

Before discussing some of the approaches that can be used to assess reflection in a written format, it is appropriate to consider some of the issues associated with this form of assessment. In general, it is acknowledged in educational circles that some students 'take to' academic writing more easily than others. This is particularly pertinent in reflective writing because the ability to express oneself clearly and concisely is a skill that is particularly important in written reflection; Wong *et al.* (1995) recognised that students' writing may not be indicative of their actual reflective abilities. Reflection is a skill that does not easily lend itself to quantifiable research methods and the correlation between written and actual reflective ability remains unknown. The beauty of reflective writing is that it enables the student to relate everyday practice to theoretical learning.

Reflective learning contract

The reflective learning contract has been used extensively to facilitate learning from practice. Very often, teachers have found that the learning contract can be the 'public face' of a student's private reflective journal and this has its drawbacks. Students have found that they cannot distinguish relevant from irrelevant material, find it difficult to include the aspect of reflection that they feel they should include, and become rather introspective (Schutz *et al.* 1996). Bolton (2010) proposed that formally assessed learning contracts lead to students following 'rules' of how to do it and also inappropriate levels of disclosure. She highlighted the important challenge of encouraging students to draw upon their journals or diaries rather than divulging raw reflection. The consequence of not doing this is that students concentrate on the descriptive and emotional aspects of events to the detriment of the evaluative (Rolfe *et al.* 2001). The challenge for the educator is how to move students on to a higher level of reflection and, as Fund *et al.* (2002) found, this is about moving to a more deliberate form of reflection, which Fund *et al.* term '*critical bridging*' (p.491). At its most effective, students use the learning contract as a dialogue with the mentor and write in it regularly, asking the mentor for written feedback. As a format for demonstrating reflective growth, the learning contract cannot be bettered for documenting practice-based reflection. At worst, it is time consuming and cumbersome. Subsequently pressures related to resources, principally the precious time of qualified nursing staff, can impact negatively on the practical use of the learning contract, particularly for pre-registration undergraduate students.

Critical incident analyses

The use of the critical incident analysis is not new; it was used initially by pilots who analysed flying missions with the intention of improving their performance (Flannigan 1954). Since then, Smith and Russell (1991),

Norman *et al.* (1992) and Perry (1997) have described the critical incident analysis as an appropriate strategy in nursing. The technique enables students to utilise a real event from practice that they can recall as having an impact on them. This may have been a positive or a negative impact. The event may be discrete, with a clear beginning and end, or more general with a variety of issues arising (Norman *et al.* 1992). When using this approach, I have found that it is important to give students guidance on the process and product of the exercise so that they are clear about what is wanted; Smith and Russell (1991) provide a useful framework, which I have slightly adapted.

1. Give a concise description of the incident, highlighting the major events.
2. Outline why you chose the event and how and why it is significant to you in both personal and professional terms.
3. Identify the key issues and why they are important.
4. Reflect on:
   - how you were involved, what you felt about the events and your part in them and why
   - why you behaved in the way you did and how you made your decisions
   - the part that others played and why you think they behaved as they did
   - what else was happening in the context at the time – were there any influential circumstances?
   - the relevant theoretical background – how were events informed by theory? what role did formal and informal theory play in the decisions made?
   - what action might be indicated either now or in the future
   - how you evaluate what happened in terms of what you have learned in a specific and in a general sense.

The specific benefits of such a tool are that it can have quite formalised guidelines, allowing students to relate the practical to the theoretical and recognise the context of the situation. These factors can help the novice and also allow the experienced reflective practitioner to create more depth in reflection. Additionally, the process of assessment is easier to conduct.

Reflective essay

The traditional essay as an assessment form is easily recognised. Such well-developed approaches can be modified effectively to assess reflective learning. The basic structure of the essay remains the same, but students are asked to write from a more personal standpoint, in the first person. This makes the student's own involvement explicit and allows exploration of practice using a reflective framework. An example of the title for a reflective essay might be: 'Reflect on and analyse the nurse's role in discharge planning in a multiprofessional setting'.

When marking a reflective essay, some of the usual 'rules' of academic writing need to be put aside. I have already mentioned that it would be written in the first person, and the assessor would be looking for evidence of personal and professional growth; this may mean that students need to include personal thought and self-disclosure. The basic academic rules remain, such as structure, referencing and critique, but there are subtle differences. Grading criteria used to assess the work would need to embrace the reflective element and give due credit for it. This is where levels of reflection can be useful; by aligning these with grading criteria, teachers can be more specific about what is wanted at each stage and engender a developmental approach to assessing reflection.

Reflective journal or diary

Using a reflective journal is, as Sylvina Tate points out in Chapter 3, a good starting point in reflective practice. Keeping a diary preserves regular time and space for reflection in a busy life. By writing about our practice experience, we can more readily articulate the subtleties of what we do and this is a valuable skill. The notion of assessing students' reflective diaries, however, is a problematic one. One of the difficulties in assessing diaries or journals is the very individuality of these; grading criteria would be very difficult to construct and utilise unless this too is individual, as Burnard (1988) suggested. Additionally, equity in marking would be a real issue. Students' reflective journals should be private, unless the student chooses to share the content at a tutorial, group meeting or in written work – importantly, this is entirely their choice. In this way, a reflective diary is an essential part of the assessment of reflection, but is not the actual vehicle for it. However, as a resource, the diary is invaluable.

Kember *et al.* (2008) suggested that students are so highly assessment driven that to remove journals from the assessment process means that they are unlikely to be kept. In my experience, it is often clear whether students use a diary, because the very act of writing a diary as the first stage in reflecting on an incident helps to sort out the relevant detail from the irrelevant. Therefore, students who keep a reflective diary and base assessed work on it are likely to achieve a higher level of reflection.

Kember *et al.* (2008) advocated the acquisition of feedback on reflective journal entries, but this does not need to be assessed. It could be an informal arrangement between students, with a personal tutor, colleague or mentor and still be as effective, without the burden of achieving certain criteria for assessment. Making this slightly more formal arrangement, as Kember *et al.* suggested, may be a useful approach but may not be so very far from formal assessment in the student's eyes. It is vital that teachers indicate to students where the assessment points are and the nature of the assessment to be carried out.

Reflective case studies

Reflective case studies are useful in allowing students to make a start at reflection, within a structured format. Often, an additional framework is used, such as a nursing model. An assignment utilising this approach might ask a student to:'Choose one aspect of care, explore the evidence base for practice and critically analyse the nursing management for a patient requiring this care. Reflect on how the nursing management of the problem could have been improved'.

This type of assessment enables the student to make meaningful connections between real-life practice and theoretical material. It also allows a personal approach, such that students can explore their own practice, as well as that of others. It would usually take the form of an academic piece of writing, although more creative and inclusive strategies could be used to present the case study, such as a presentation or poster.

Reflective portfolio

Portfolios are a statutory requirement for nurses and for this reason seem to be a useful way of assessing reflection in the long term. There is considerable and growing support for the use of reflective portfolios in education and this has become a popular strategy in nursing courses. The portfolio would be a collection of evidence and reflection on that evidence, to demonstrate progression in reflection over time. The advantages of the use of a portfolio to assess reflection are that:

● it can incorporate evidence of many different forms of reflection – individual, group, written and verbal
● it is self-directed – a key skill for reflection
● it can be built upon over time – indeed, it is based on this premise
● it allows students to work at their own reflective level.

However, there are some issues in using portfolios to assess reflection and these include the relative advantage that some students with certain learning styles may have (this is a common issue with assessment in general), the time-consuming nature of the work involved in gathering evidence and the prescriptive form that portfolios can take. Recently, the use of online learning has begun to stimulate the development of e-portfolios that students put together online.

Grading reflection

Although levels of reflection are widely covered in the literature in relation to depth or progression, the association of these levels with assessment has not been further explored. It appears that in many of these descriptors of progression, higher-level reflection embraces broader issues than just what is happening immediately around the student, to include application of theory to practice and a change in the student's perspective. Mezirow (1991) generated a seven-level descriptor of reflective progression, which, although highly theoretical, is nonetheless useful.

Smith and Hatton (1995) describe three levels of reflection, which move from descriptive to dialogic to critical. Conversely, Richardson (1995) introduces a way of seeing reflective development as multifaceted and not linear or hierarchical. This has some face value, considering that it is clear that some students have a greater potential for reflective practice than others. It allows for a more individual and inclusive approach with multiple 'entry' and 'exit' points. Unfortunately, it is a difficult conceptual model to translate into assessment criteria. Nevertheless, one should try to assess students' starting points individually, and recognise that some progress more quickly and further than others.

Issues for students and teaching staff in the assessment of reflection

The difficulties that staff and students find in the assessment of reflection mirror the broader problems. A study by Angove (1999) explored the perspectives of academic staff in the assessment of reflection, finding that they held equivocal views of what they were actually assessing. A major area of concern was about the correlation between good reflective writing and its translation into practice; this is echoed by other authors (for example, Stewart and Richardson 2000). Also, some staff were not clear about how grading criteria related to levels of reflection and this influenced the guidance that students received.

There are a number of issues here that may have a negative impact on the reliability of an assessment tool and it is clear that agreed values, consistent support and feedback and adequate preparation of staff assessing reflection are important. These issues are congruent with the findings of Stewart and Richardson (2000) who explored the experiences of occupational therapy and physiotherapy students. In this study both staff and students had reservations about the assessment of reflection and again, levels of support for students varied. Following their findings, Stewart and Richardson proposed more of a focus on the *process* of reflection, rather than the outcomes. This gives some support to the use of levels of reflection and to the use of self-assessment in order to move students through the levels.

King and Kitchener (1994) developed a model of reflective judgement from their work with college students. They suggested that the student's ability to manage their college work depends partly on the recognition that issues can be ill defined and demand reflective judgement. In fact, we as nurses would recognise this in practice – we just need to translate the understanding into reflecting on the process of reflection. Of course, this echoes the original work of Schön (1983, 1987) who described these aspects of professional practice as the 'swampy lowlands'. King and Kitchener's model has seven stages in which assumptions about the nature of knowledge increase in sophistication with accompanying development of the ability to reflect on poorly structured situations.

Pre-reflective stages

Stage one: Knowledge is absolute
Stage two: Knowledge is absolute but not always immediately available
Stage three: Knowledge is absolute in the majority of cases, but briefly uncertain in others

Quasi-reflective stages

Stage four: Knowledge is uncertain, as there is always a constituent of ambiguity in evidence
Stage five: Knowledge is personal, since individuals must interpret the evidence

Reflective stages

Stage six: Knowledge concerning ill-structured problems is constructed by appraising other's evidence
Stage seven: Knowledge of ill-structured problems is constructed from inquiry, which leads to sensible solutions based on currently available evidence

This model has some potential for dealing with negative experiences of staff and students in the assessment of reflection. King and Kitchener (1994) suggest that first-year students could be expected to be at level three to four, whilst senior students could be expected to be at level four. Thus a qualifying nurse may only reach the quasi-reflective stage at entry to primary practice. This may be a useful means of overcoming the fear that many experienced practitioners have of reflection, as so many cannot see their own inherent reflective abilities when they are asked to engage in reflection or feel that they are engaging in reflection when they are not. In formal courses, linking this to grading criteria may be useful but, more importantly, the model could be used to help both assessors and students to come to terms with the ambiguities and lack of definition in what is being assessed.

What assessors and teachers of reflection need to come to terms with is the fact that their role is 'guide on the side' rather than 'sage on the stage' (Durgahee 1998). Thus teachers and assessors are facilitators rather than anything else. Facilitation is, supposedly, widely accepted in nurse education, yet it seems likely that this less than distinct role is actually what is causing the problems here. Teachers are often asked to be both facilitators and assessors of reflection and this can cause tensions at best and conflict at worst.

Evaluating reflection

As reflection has become integrated within nurse education, it is increasingly important to demonstrate the benefits for professional practice and health and social care delivery. It is only through effective evaluation that this impact can be quantified. It is argued that all educational activity needs evaluation (Herbener and Watson 1992), and indeed as students and educators, it is a large part of our daily lives. With the growing use of reflection in both pre- and postregistration programmes over the past decade, evaluation of this approach is well overdue. Whilst reflection is perceived to play a key role in the development of effective practitioners of nursing, there is a lack of empirical evidence to support the assertion that engaging in reflective practice actually changes or in any way benefits patient care. The situated, contextually bound benefits to practice that may result from reflective practice cannot often be labelled as 'clinically effective'.

Thus, evaluating reflection and reflective practice needs to be seen more in context. How can a nurse's development in practice, as an outcome of reflective activity, be measured? Whilst reflective assessments as part of an overall assessment strategy can be quantified using grading systems, such as those described above, this alone is not sufficient. We need to address the pervasive anxiety about whether good reflective writing equals good reflective practice. Writing about practice development as a result of reflection may not equate with actual practice development as we have seen, let alone be a direct consequence of reflection. We must also recognise that measuring the practice development of an individual is fraught with difficulties, as so many other variables may have an influence. As Heath (1998) points out, reflection as a concept does not lend itself to the research approaches that can make such a measurement anyway.

As a first step, it is useful to consider the potential outcomes of reflection, as this will help to inform potential evaluation criteria. Boud *et al.* (1985) suggested that the outcomes of reflection are both cognitive and affective in nature, providing a list of potential outcomes summarised into four key areas.

1. New perspectives on experience
2. Change in behaviour
3. Readiness for application
4. Commitment to action

Chapter 8

Reflective learning, then, may be evaluated by measuring the extent to which a student has a changed perspective on practice as a result of experience. This change in perspective may also lead to changes in attitudes, values and consequently behaviour. The learner should demonstrate motivation to apply new knowledge and skills in practice. There may also be a deepening of understanding of their own learning style and needs, with a positive attitude towards further learning. Reflection should be a journey that spirals into deeper reflection; see Chapter7 for Sue Duke's ongoing and fascinating experience of this and you will see how measuring the outcomes of reflection may not be a straightforward activity. Boud *et al.* (1985) recognised that some of these outcomes are intangible and may not be easily demonstrated or observed in the practice completion of an educational programme. Thus, questions emerge about the most effective strategy for accurately measuring outcomes of reflection and therefore for evaluating its success.

Whilst the issue of evaluating reflective learning is recognised in the literature, a limited number of studies have been conducted in this area. Strategies that can be utilised include:

- qualitative evaluation by assessors and students
- surveys collecting quantitative evaluation data
- meta-analysis of data from student assessments of a reflective nature
- qualitative and quantitative evaluation of student performance in a reflective practice setting where students are placed.

The main focus of this type of evaluation is to find the degree to which there is a change in a student or practitioner's action as a demonstration of new knowledge or new skills. The key issue in terms of approach is to ask and also observe, so that what is espoused and what is actually present in practice are both evaluated.

Exploration is likely to be made around the following criteria.

1. Development of the knowledge base
2. Development of new skills or the advancement of previous skills
3. A change in or refining of attitudes and values
4. Participation in reflective activities
5. Clinical practice development initiatives

This approach relies heavily on individual perceptions of development in practice and this may not be an effective method of evaluation due to interrater reliability issues. Utilising exemplars from practice to illustrate the measurement of criteria above can contribute towards the veracity of findings much as the use of participants' own words does in qualitative research. Approaches such as fourth-generation evaluation (Guba and Lincoln 1989) may be a valuable way in which to consider evaluation of reflection. This strategy utilises the methodology of qualitative inquiry to collect and evaluate data from the perspectives of stakeholders (those experiencing the phenomenon). This would include patients, families, nursing staff, students, medical and allied health professionals, facilitators and mentors.

Andrews *et al.* (1998) asserted that patient outcomes should be included in evaluating reflective practice to determine if the benefits of reflection are transmitted to patient outcomes. Without this, the cycle is not complete, although this is likely to be some time coming. Durgahee (1998) suggested that patients' perceptions of reflective practitioners should be included in evaluation of reflective practice – that would be a truly interesting study. Research of this nature, although needed, demands some considerable skill of a researcher and there would need to be robust research strategies in place to achieve this. Yet Rome was not built in a day and less sophisticated areas need attention before we are ready to approach this one. The need to evaluate the benefits of reflection is closely allied to the need to evaluate how it is facilitated and assessed. There are some particular imperatives.

- The need to identify strategies which will map change in practice over time as a result of reflective practice, as distinct from other variables.
- How to include patient perspectives in the evaluation.
- The need for long-term studies which will elicit the effects of reflection on practitioners over time.

It is clearly very important that where reflection is assessed, the relative merits of assessment strategies, and their levels of success, are evaluated. In the earlier parts of this chapter, evaluation and assessment were defined as being two distinct activities, but it is clearly the case that, where one is attempted, the other must be too. Evaluation of an assessment strategy must involve both placing a relative value on it and also measuring its success.

Conclusion

In this chapter I have debated what is meant by the terms 'assessment' and 'evaluation' in relation to reflection. Definitions have been put forward and the contextual issues discussed. I have highlighted some of the philosophical issues that arise when attempting to assess reflection and offered a perspective on these. The challenges associated with assessment of reflection have been indicated and some practical solutions suggested. Tools that are available for assessment are outlined, with a discussion of some of the relative benefits and issues. The evaluation of reflective practice is also discussed and some research priorities offered.

In summary, reflective practice is a means to enhance effective interventions with patients and clients in nursing. Reflection is therefore central

Chapter 8

to nurse education and must be treated as such. This involves making clear and unambiguous assessment of the abilities of those engaged in reflection and working at developing these over time. Evaluating the efficacy of these strategies is vital in order to instigate change and progress the art and science of reflective practice.

References

Andrews, M., Gidman, J. and Humphreys, A. (1998) Reflection: does it enhance professional nursing practice? *British Journal of Nursing*, **7**(7), 413–417.

Angove, C.J. (1999) Lecturer and lecturer practitioners' perceptions of grading students' reflection on experience in learning contracts. Unpublished MSc thesis, University of Manchester.

Ashford, D., Blake, D., Knott, C., Platzer, H. and Snelling, J. (1998) Changing conceptions of reflective practice in social work, health and education. An institutional case study. *Journal of Interprofessional Care*, **12**(1), 7–19.

Bolton, G. (2010) *Reflective Practice. Writing and Professional Development*, 3rd edn. Sage, London.

Boud, D., Keogh, R. and Walker, D. (eds) (1985) *Reflection: Turning Experience into Learning*. Kogan Pag, London.

Burnard, P. (1988) The journal as an assessment tool in nurse education. *Nurse Education Today*, **8**, 105–107.

Burrows, D.E. (1995) The nurse teacher's role in the promotion of reflective practice. *Nurse Education Today*, **15**, 346–350.

Burton, A.J. (2000) Reflection: nursing's practice and education panacea? *Journal of Advanced Nursing*, **31**(5), 1009–1017.

Cotton, A.H. (2001) Private thoughts in the public sphere: issues in reflection and reflective practice in nursing. *Journal of Advanced Nursing*, **36**(4), 512–519.

Daly, W. (1998) Critical thinking as an outcome of nursing education, what is it? Why is it important to nursing practice? *Journal of Advanced Nursing*, **28**, 323–331.

Duffy, A. (2008). Guiding students through reflective practice – the preceptors' experiences. A qualitative descriptive study. *Nursing Education in Practice*, **9**(3), 166–175.

Durgahee, T. (1998) Facilitating reflection: from a sage on a stage to a guide on the side. *Nurse Education Today*, **18**, 158–164.

Eraut, M. (1994) *Developing Professional Knowledge and Competence*. Routledge Falmer, London.

Flannigan, J.C. (1954) The critical incident technique. *Psychological Bulletin*, **51**, 327–358.

Fund, Z., Court, D. and Kramarski, B. (2002) Construction and application of an evaluative tool to assess reflection in teacher-training courses. *Assessment and Evaluation in Higher Education*, **27**(6), 481–499.

Getliffe, K.A. (1996) An examination of the use of reflection in the assessment of practice for undergraduate nursing students. *International Journal of Nursing Studies*, **33**(4), 361–374.

Ghaye, Y. and Lillyman, S. (2010) *Reflection: Principles and Practice for Health Care Professionals*. Quay Books, London.

Gibbs, G., Farmer, B. and Eastcott, D. (1988) *Learning by Doing. A Guide to Teaching and Learning Methods*. Far Eastern University, Birmingham Polytechnic, Birmingham.

Glaze, J.E. (2002) Stages in coming to terms with reflection: student advanced nurse practitioners' perceptions of their reflective journeys. *Journal of Advanced Nursing*, **37**(30), 265–272.

Goodman, J. (1984) Reflection and teacher education: a case study and theoretical analysis. *Interchange*, **15**(3), 9–26.

Guba, E.G. and Lincoln, D.Y.S. (1989) *Fourth Generation Evaluation*. Sage, California.

Hannigan, B. (2001) A discussion of the strengths and weaknesses of 'reflection' in nursing practice and education. *Journal of Clinical Nursing*, **10**, 278–283.

Heath, H. (1998) Reflection and patterns of knowing in nursing. *Journal of Advanced Nursing*, **27**, 1054–1059.

Herbener, D. and Watson, J. (1992) Models for evaluating nurse education programmes. *Nursing Outlook*, **40**(1), 27–32.

Johns, C. and Freshwater, D. (2009) *Transforming Nursing Through Reflective Practice*, 3rd edn. Blackwell Science, Oxford.

Kember, D. Jones, A. Loke, A.Y., *et al.* (2008) Encouraging reflective writing. In: Kember, D. (ed) *Reflective Teaching and Learning in the Health Professions*, 2nd edn. Blackwell Science, Oxford.

King, P.M. and Kitchener, K.S. (1994) *Developing Reflective Judgement: Understanding and Promoting Intellectual Growth and Critical Thinking in Adolescents and Adults*. Jossey-Bass, San Francisco.

Korthagen, F.A.J. and Wubbels, T. (1995) Characteristics of reflective practitioners: towards an operationalisation of the concept of reflection. *Teachers and Teaching: Theory and Practice*, **1**(1), 51–72.

Mallik, M. (1998) The role of nurse educators in the development of reflective practitioners: a selective case study of the Australian and UK experience. *Nurse Education Today*, **18**(1), 52–63.

McCarthy, B. and Murphy, S. (2008) Assessing undergraduate nursing students in clinical practice: do preceptors use assessment strategies? *Nurse Education Today*, **28**(3), 301–313.

Mezirow, J. (1991) *Transformative Dimensions of Adult Learning*. Jossey-Bass, San Francisco.

Morgan, R. and Johns, C. (2009) The beast and the star: resolving contradictions in everyday practice. In: Johns, C. (ed) *Transforming Nursing Through Reflective Practice*, 2nd edn. Blackwell, Oxford.

Newell, R. (1994) Reflection: art, science or pseudo-science? (Editorial) *Nurse Education Today*, **14**, 79–81.

Norman, I., Redfern, S., Tomalin, D. and Oliver, S. (1992) Developing Flannigan's critical incident technique to elicit indicators of high and low quality nursing care from patients and their nurses. *Journal of Advanced Nursing*, **17**, 590–600.

Paget, T. (2001) Reflective practice and clinical outcomes: practitioners' views on how reflective practice has influenced their clinical practice. *Journal of Clinical Nursing*, **10**, 204–214.

Chapter 8

Perry, L. (1997) Critical incidents, crucial issues: insights into the working lives of registered nurses. *Journal of Clinical Nursing*, **6**, 131–137.

Phillips, T., Schostak, J. and Tyler, J. (2000) *Practice and Assessment in Nursing and Midwifery: Doing it for Real*. English National Board for Nursing, Midwifery and Health Visiting, Researching Professional Education Series. English National Board for Nursing, Midwifery and Health Visiting, London.

Platzer, H., Blake, D. and Ashford, D. (2000a) Barriers to learning from reflection: a study of the use of group-work with post-registration nurses. *Journal of Advanced Nursing*, **31**(5), 1001–1008.

Platzer, H., Blake, D. and Ashford, D. (2000b) An evaluation of process and outcomes form learning through reflective practice groups on a post-registration nursing course. *Journal of Advanced Nursing*, **31**(3), 689–695

Reece-Jones, P. (1995) Hindsight bias in reflective practice: an empirical investigation *Journal of Advanced Nursing*, **21**(4), 783–788.

Rich, A. and Parker, D. (1995) Reflection and critical incident analysis: ethical and moral implications of their use within nursing and midwifery education. *Journal of Advanced Nursing*, **22**, 1050–1057.

Richardson, R. (1995) Humpty Dumpty: reflection and reflective nursing practice. *Journal of Advanced Nursing*, **21**, 1044–1050.

Rolfe, G., Freshwater, D., and Jasper, M. (2001) *Critical Reflection for Nursing and the Helping Professions*. Palgrave, Basingstoke.

Schön, D. (1983) *The Reflective Practitioner*. Jossey-Bass, San Francisco.

Schön, D.A. (1987) *Educating the Reflective Practitioner*. Jossey-Bass, San Francisco.

Schutz, S., Bulman, C. and Salussolia, M. (1996) The learning contract as a tool for documenting competence. *Teaching News (Oxford Brookes University)*, **43**, 17–18.

Smith, A. and Russell, J. (1991) Using critical incidents in nurse education *Nurse Education Today*, **11**(4), 284–291.

Smith, N. and Hatton, D. (1995) Reflection in teacher education. *Towards definition and implementation. Teaching and Teacher Education*, **11**(1), 33–49.

Stewart, S. and Richardson, B. (2000) Reflection and its place in the curriculum: should it be assessed? *Assessment and Evaluation in Higher Education*, **25**(4), 369–380.

Sumison, J. and Fleet, A. (1996) Reflection: can we assess it? *Assessment and Evaluation in Higher Education*, **21**(2), 121–130.

Valli, L. (1993) Reflective teacher education programs: an analysis of case studies In: Calderhead, J. and Gates, P. (eds) *Conceptualising Reflection in Teacher Development*. Falmer Press, London.

Van Horn, R. and Freed, S. (2008) Journaling and dialogue pairs to promote reflection in clinical nursing education. *Nursing Education Perspectives*, **29**(4), 220–225.

Wong, F., Kember, D., Chung, L. and Yan, L. (1995) Assessing the level of student reflection from reflective journals. *Journal of Advanced Nursing*, **22**, 48–57.

Chapter 9

Getting started on a journey with reflection

Chris Bulman

Faculty of Health and Life Sciences, Oxford Brookes University, Oxford, UK

Contemplating the journey

At the start of a journey with reflection, the path might not be apparent straight away. My experience with reflection, and facilitating its use in students and colleagues, tells me that most people are relieved to be offered some words of encouragement as well as some very practical help. I believe that talking with others who have some experience of using reflection and being given a few handy hints can boost people's confidence with the whole process. Also, artful teachers recognise the need to support students in new ways of thinking and learning about their practice, whilst realising that critically reflecting on your practice is not an easy journey. Reflection is something that needs to be worked at, it is something that requires time and commitment. Reflection can be painful and frustrating; it can be surprising and eye-opening. It can be, as Sue Duke describes in Chapter 7, 'a big ask'. Yet, despite critiques in the literature (e.g. Burnard 2005), I believe that reflection can be an extremely valuable way to learn from experience and so to challenge practice. Here is a final chapter to boost your confidence in 'getting started on your journey'.

Just as in life, nursing involves situations that are complex. Schön (1983) has described this as the 'swampy lowlands' of practice problems; it can be messy and chaotic. If you want to understand nursing and yourself as a nurse, you need to try and make sense of the complexity and reflection can help you to do this. The important point here is that reflection is not just about learning in the traditional academic sense but really is an investment in learning about yourself as a nurse, and also by the way as a person, since you don't stop being a person as soon as you put on a uniform. The journey should begin with the realisation that we bring ourselves to our practice, to every situation that we encounter, however much the past traditions of nursing, and current narrow interpretations of evidence-based practice, have encouraged us not to do so.

Having, and drawing on, a repertoire of experience

Having a repertoire of experience is useful for the purposes of reflection and can help to inform clinical judgement. As Schön suggested (1987), we can then draw on experiences, make comparisons and recognise when things do not fit. It is possible to use the difficult, uncomfortable and surprising moments of practice to grow as practitioners because, through reflection, it is possible to learn and move on from these experiences (Bulman and Schutz 2007). (Don't forget that there is also value in using positive experiences for reflective purposes as well as the negative.) Nursing knowledge from your practice repertoire and from life experiences can easily be undervalued as simple and ordinary. Yet, actively learning from our experiences can be one of the most valuable ways of developing self and practice, so I want to encourage you to appreciate that developing a repertoire of experience is important.

Having a repertoire of experience is logically associated with experienced practitioners. I know from my own teaching and research that experienced practitioners definitely do draw on this wealth of experience as they develop their reflection. However, there is a point of view suggesting that reflection is not so helpful in the education of pre-registration undergraduates who by virtue of their situation have little or no experience of nursing (Powell 1998). This does not mean that if you are a new student you should discount the practice of reflection. I want to inspire you to think about the experiences you already have. You may not have huge amounts of professional experience but nevertheless, the life experiences you bring to your professional programme can be very positively used. You may have suffered a loss, gone through childbirth, had a hospital stay or had dealings with a variety of healthcare professionals. Think about how much you have already learnt about yourself, how others react to you, what you value about life, love and health before you even set foot inside a university or a clinical area as a student. You bring all of this as a gift when reflecting on your professional practice and can slowly begin to build up reflective skills which hopefully then extend over a lifetime.

Most importantly, I would like to encourage you to nurture a sense of wonder about practice, to grow and learn through your practice, rather than rely on ritual and habit to get you through the day. Eisner (1991) has suggested that we simply do not use what we have no immediate use for; indeed, when we are new to something this may often be the case – we simply do not see everything we might. Lack of experience, knowledge and judgement can lead to incomplete or limited understandings of practice. However, with encouragement, over time and with judicial use of reflection, it is possible to develop what Eisner calls an 'enlightened eye', where through our experience we can develop meaning, abilities and values rather than just merely looking and thus we can begin to see the world in a different way.

If a repertoire of practice is to be in any way useful, we need to value and communicate it. With the right support as well as challenge, reflection has the potential to ease and open up dialogue and provide a language with which to express our practice to others. As a profession, we need to be more proud and confident of this personal and professional knowing since it offers a wealth of understanding and ability to make sense of practice. The following interview extract (Bulman 2009) shows Alison, an experienced practitioner and nurse educator, talking about writing a piece of reflection for the first time.

> ... a day or two later I went back to what I had written and it just made such an impact on me. I thought, oh my God! I worked in palliative care all these years, I have never written down what I had done with people in this real profound work that you do with people at the end of their lives and it was just such a powerful thing to read! And I suppose that was the turning point for me in terms of reflection – it became something that had made an impact on me.

This extract demonstrates the importance of having, and drawing on, a repertoire of experience. It captures a sense of the potential of reflection to liberate the knowledge that we have as nurses and that is often taken for granted.

Reflection, change and challenge

Effective practice needs to be focused and goal directed and therefore reflection cannot just be concerned with understanding, but must locate practice within its social and political structures (Bolton 2005) and its role in changing practice (Driscoll 2007). To achieve this, reflective development needs the right culture, one that is conducive to open inquiry, support and challenge and one based on practice, with theory generated from and related to practice (Mantzoukas and Jasper 2004). This assumes that people want to strive for change and are not content with their 'lot'. It also raises the point that encouraging individuals to develop reflection may be a way of diverting organisational responsibilities for developing practice onto the wonderfully broad shoulders of practitioners – something to reflect on!

I also want to highlight that 'moving on' in your practice, as a result of reflection, is not always easy since it takes courage and commitment to change and take action. The outcome of reflection may be about you changing as an individual but it may also mean deciding to take action as a team or organisation. Listening to other practitioners has confirmed my own experiences that changing one's own practice may be easier than encouraging a team or organisation to take action. In addition, the freedom to question and challenge does not always exist and circumstances may dictate that it is easier to leave well alone than to challenge the status quo. These issues need to be considered, because change can be slow or even impossible sometimes and also because reflection might simply result in the affirmation of an idea or experience rather than in any immediately perceivable change. Cynicism aside, change and development are possible through reflection especially where it is supported by colleagues and by the culture within which people work (Smith and Gray 2001; Clouder and Sellars 2004). However, these issues are worth contemplating in true reflective style.

Another careful word is justified at this point. Although I believe that reflection offers most of us a positive route for exploring therapeutic practice (practice that makes a difference to patients), this can only be achieved by nurturing self-awareness and constructive criticality. This has consequences since reflection is not always comfortable; this is a point amply illustrated throughout this book. Critical reflection will mean facing incongruity, uncertainty and uncomfortable facts about yourself, nursing and the health services you work in. You need to consider how you will deal with both the positive and negative aspects before embarking on a reflective pathway. Organisations have a responsibility to provide suitable support and challenge if they want to nurture reflective practitioners. Moreover, educationalists introducing reflection as part of a curriculum need to be aware of this and carefully consider the support required for such an approach.

The important points that arise from contemplating a journey with reflection are summarised below.

- Reflection can be a valuable way to learn from experience and challenge practice.
- Reflection provides a means by which you can critically consider how practice affects you and how you affect practice.
- Reflection is helped by dialogue – it requires both support and challenge.
- Reflection should be connected with change and action.
- Nursing problems can be complex and messy.
- Changing practice and self is not always easy.
- Reflection is not always comfortable and requires time and commitment.
- Developing a repertoire of experience is important for reflection and can inform clinical judgement.
- Nursing knowledge is important and is often undervalued.
- Reflection can liberate knowledge that we take for granted and can help us to develop an 'enlightened eye'.
- Nurses need to grow and learn through their practice in order to develop as therapeutic practitioners and reflection can offer a positive

route to explore therapeutic nursing (nursing that makes a difference to patients).

- Practice and education organisations have a role to play in the development of reflective nursing.

Key suggestions for your journey with reflection

Some of the suggestions mentioned below will seem familiar, as they have been covered in different contexts throughout the book. They are either represented here in a summarised form or developed a little further in order to give you the chance to consider what you need to work on, without needing to plough through the book, except where you require some further detail. It is worth considering:

- working on your skills for reflection
- using a framework to help you to reflect
- finding someone to reflect with
- developing your reflective writing
- reading some of the literature
- having the courage to change and challenge.

Working on your skills for reflection

Developing your skills for reflection is essential. Chapter 2 provides a comprehensive look at the skills we believe are essential for you to successfully develop your reflection. Additionally, if you are a teacher, Chapter 2 will remind you about what you could 'stitch in' to your curriculum in order to help your students with the development of their skills. The skills are presented here in a summarised form in Box 9.1.

More help with critical analysis

Critical analysis involves separation of a whole into its component parts and detailed examination of those parts, in order to make judgements about the strengths and weaknesses of the different parts as well as the whole. Using a metaphor here is helpful. Imagine yourself knocking down a brick wall – you stand there mallet in hand and gaze at it purposefully. At this stage it is just a pile of bricks in need of demolition. You knock it to the ground and now you start to see things that you had not noticed before – the crumbling mortar that held it together, various tiny creatures that had made it their home, the odd bit of graffiti, the posters that someone had stuck on it. And, of course, the individual bricks! The point here is that through looking a little closer, you can began to see the different parts that made up your wall as well as the whole.

Box 9.1   Skills for reflection

Self-awareness	Analysis of feelings. Involves an exploration of how a situation has affected you and how you have affected a situation
Description	Ability to recognise and recollect accurately relevant events and key features of an experience and to give a comprehensive account of the situation
Critical analysis	Examining the components of a situation, identifying existing knowledge, challenging assumptions and imagining and exploring alternatives. You can use critical analysis of knowledge to weigh up how relevant such knowledge may be to a particular situation you are reflecting on
Synthesis	Integration of new knowledge with previous knowledge. You can use synthesis in a creative way to solve problems and to predict likely consequences of actions
Evaluation	Evaluation encourages you to make a judgement about the value of something. Synthesis and evaluation are crucial in the development of new perspectives

The skill of critical analysis is not easy so don't lose heart if you don't get it straight away; use your mentor/supervisor/tutor to help you. In summary, it involves the following activities.

● Identifying existing knowledge relevant to the situation
● Exploring feelings about the situation and the influence of these
● Identifying and challenging assumptions made
● Imagining and exploring other courses of action

More help with synthesis

Synthesis involves building up ideas into a connected and coherent whole; it is about original thinking and creativity (think about how you would build up a brand new wall!). Synthesis in reflective practice involves integration of new knowledge, feelings or attitudes with previous knowledge, feelings or attitudes; it leads to a fresh insight or new perspective on practice.

Some useful frameworks for reflection

You may be filled with enthusiasm about reflection but the dilemma of where to start is common. Frameworks help with going about the business of reflection. It may be that you feel comfortable with one particular framework and opt to use it every time you reflect. Whilst experience tells me they are valued by novices, it is not essential to use a framework; some people choose not to. It is worth highlighting Johns' (2000) caution that frameworks are just devices to help you with reflection, they are not designed to impose a prescription of what reflection is. Bolton (2005) has made the point that frameworks can be as much about control as guidance and therefore they should be viewed and used with these critiques in mind. Also, whilst some may not overtly promote a critical theory approach (see Chapter 1), they do at least guide the user to think about critiquing experience for future action and the influences and consequences of action. The suggestions below are not exhaustive; there are more available in the literature.

Gibbs' Reflective Cycle (adapted and updated from Gibbs *et al.* 1988, pp.46–47)

When we first started to develop the use of reflection at Oxford Brookes University (then Oxford Polytechnic) towards the end of the 1980s, we were keen to find a user-friendly framework that would help everyone with the process. Then everyone was a beginner with reflection, teachers and mentors as well as students, so drawing from Gibbs' work on experiential learning proved to be extremely helpful. Graham Gibbs worked at Oxford Polytechnic at the time so we drew on his expertise and were lead to a book on experiential learning he had produced with a project team from the then Birmingham Polytechnic called *Learning by Doing* (Gibbs *et al.* 1988). Several years on, students as well as staff still find the Reflective Cycle of value and we have adapted and updated it recently to develop a more user-friendly tool.

The Reflective Cycle originally draws on the work of Kolb (1984) in order to explain how people can learn from their experience. Kolb's work on learning from experience suggested the utility of using practice in order to develop and test out theory. This emphasises the importance of drawing on the wealth of experience students inevitably bring to their education and continue to develop over a lifetime. The Reflective Cycle as currently used at Oxford Brookes University has been updated and adapted from Gibbs' original cycle of structured debriefing following an experience. This process was recommended by Gibbs because discussions or debriefings can so easily 'lurch from superficial descriptions of what happened to premature conclusions about what to do next, without adequate reflection or analysis.' (p.46). Significantly, Gibbs emphasised the requirement to deal with both *description of events* and *feelings* in order to be able to move on to the implications and action plans that arise from an experience reflected upon. These were important considerations that resonated with me and my colleagues as we have learnt about reflection, used it and facilitated it in others.

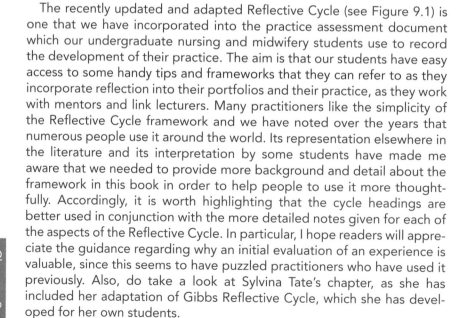

Figure 9.1   Reflective Cycle (Adapted and updated from Gibbs *et al.* (1988)).

The recently updated and adapted Reflective Cycle (see Figure 9.1) is one that we have incorporated into the practice assessment document which our undergraduate nursing and midwifery students use to record the development of their practice. The aim is that our students have easy access to some handy tips and frameworks that they can refer to as they incorporate reflection into their portfolios and their practice, as they work with mentors and link lecturers. Many practitioners like the simplicity of the Reflective Cycle framework and we have noted over the years that numerous people use it around the world. Its representation elsewhere in the literature and its interpretation by some students have made me aware that we needed to provide more background and detail about the framework in this book in order to help people to use it more thoughtfully. Accordingly, it is worth highlighting that the cycle headings are better used in conjunction with the more detailed notes given for each of the aspects of the Reflective Cycle. In particular, I hope readers will appreciate the guidance regarding why an initial evaluation of an experience is valuable, since this seems to have puzzled practitioners who have used it previously. Also, do take a look at Sylvina Tate's chapter, as she has included her adaptation of Gibbs Reflective Cycle, which she has developed for her own students.

Description
What happened?
- Describe what happened.
- Keep focused on your description; don't make judgements or draw conclusions.

Feelings
What were your feelings and how did you react?
- Keep focused on your emotions, don't be tempted to analyse yet.

Initial evaluation of the experience
What was good and bad about the experience?
- Evaluate your initial feelings and reactions in order to get to the heart of what really concerned you (positive or negative) about the experience. By doing this, you should be able to identify and attend to key issue/s which will allow you to move on to critical analysis.
- NB: It is important to keep focused, so try to choose just one or two issues. Then you can move on to develop some in-depth critical analysis rather than just 'skim the surface' of many.

Critical analysis
What sense did you make of the experience?
- Critically analyse what was going on. Were people's experiences similar to or different from yours, and in what ways? What themes seem to be emerging from your analysis? How do these compare with your previous experiences? Can you challenge any assumptions now?
- NB: Make use of knowledge/ideas from outside your experience to develop and inform your analysis, e.g. experts, mentors, policy, research, law and ethics, literature, clinical papers, reviews, discussion papers. How do these compare with your experience?

Conclusions
What have you learnt from reflecting on this experience?
- What have you learnt about: yourself, your self-awareness, your practice?
- What have you learnt that you would recommend for practice in general (i.e. social, political, cultural, ethical issues)?

Final evaluation and action plan
What would you do differently?
- What would you do if this type of situation arose again?
- What steps will you take, based on what you've learnt, to develop your future practice?
- How will you decide if your practice has been improved?

Chapter 9

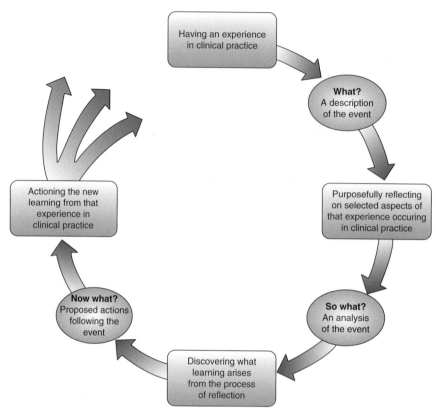

Figure 9.2   The What? Model of Structured Reflection and associated trigger questions (Based on Driscoll and O'Sullivan 2007, p.6).

The What? Model of Structured Reflection (Driscoll 2007)

John Driscoll is a nurse and lecturer and also works as a professional development consultant and coach. John is the co-author of the chapter on clinical supervision in this book. Whilst undergoing teacher training, he came up with this model when completing an assignment exploring the use of questioning. He was unaware that Borton (1970) had used similar question headings some years earlier in the USA. Driscoll's model was first published some time ago (Driscoll 1994) and he has developed this latest version which appears in Figure 9.2. It shows the pragmatic nature of his approach to reflection and is particularly strong on the action element and the requirement to make a difference, influenced by his passion for good coaching. We use a simplified version of this model with our undergraduate students when asking them to reflect on their contribution to teamwork on an interprofessional module.

1. A description of the event

What? Trigger questions

- What is the purpose of returning to this situation?
- What happened?
- What did I see/do?
- What was my reaction to it?
- What did other people do who were involved in this?

2. An analysis of the event

So What? Trigger questions

- How did I feel at the time of the event?
- Were the feelings I had any different from those of other people who were also involved at the time?
- Are my feelings now, after the event, any different from what I experienced at the time?
- Do I feel troubled; if so, in what way?
- What were the effects of what I did (or did not do)?
- What positive aspects now emerge for me from the event that happened in practice?
- What have I noticed about my behaviour in practice by taking a more measured look at it?
- What observations does any person helping me to reflect on my practice make of the way I acted at the time?

3. Proposed actions following the event Now What? Trigger questions

- What are the implications for me and others in clinical practice based on what I have described and analysed?
- What difference does it make if I choose to do nothing?
- Where can I get more information to face a similar situation again?
- How could I modify my practice if a similar situation were to happen again?
- What support do I need to help me 'action' the results of my reflections?
- Which aspect should be tackled first?
- How will I notice that I am any different in clinical practice?
- What is the main learning I take from reflecting on my practice in this way?

Model for Structured Reflection (Johns 2009)

Chris Johns' (2009) Model for Structured Reflection (MSR) is composed of a series of questions helping the reflective practitioner to tune into an experience and provides organisation and meaning to the process of reflection (Box 9.2). Significantly, the first reflective cue encourages the reflective practitioner to 'bring the mind home'. Johns (2009, p.52) has

Box 9.2   Model for Structured Reflection (Source: Johns 2009)

Reflective cue

- Bring the mind home.
- Focus on a description of an experience that seems significant in some way.
- What issues are significant to pay attention to?
- How do I interpret the way people were feeling and why they felt that way?
- How was I feeling and what made me feel that way?
- What was I trying to achieve, and did I respond effectively?
- What were the consequences of my actions on the patient, others and myself?
- What factors influence the way I was/am feeling, thinking or responding to this situation?
- What knowledge did or might have informed me?
- To what extent did I act for the best and in tune with my values?
- How does this situation connect with previous experiences?
- How might I reframe the situation and respond more effectively given this situation again?
- What would be the consequences of alternative actions for the patient, others and myself?
- What factors might constrain me responding in new ways?
- How do I NOW feel about this experience?
- Am I more able to support myself and others better as a consequence?
- What insights have I gained?
- Am I more able to realise desirable practice?

described this as a 'preparatory cue', placing a person in the 'best position to reflect'. His inspiration here comes from his study of Buddhist meditation and his 'focus on bringing the mind home helps to shift the balance of seeing reflection as a cognitive activity to a more meditative activity'. Importantly, such a focus requires time, space and an appropriate environment for reflective contemplation. Johns' chapter on 'Becoming reflective' (pp.41–79) provides more detail and examples regarding the other reflective cues in this model. Additionally, Chapter 3 in this book on reflective writing draws in more detail on other aspects of Johns' work.

Chris Johns has developed his model for structured reflection over several years, recognising the usefulness of such a technique, at least in the initial stages, to guide people with their early reflection.

'Having worked through the reflective cues, I seek to gain insights. As I become more experienced at reflection, I internalise the cues

> ### Box 9.3   Reflective Framework (Source: Stephenson 1994, pp.56–57)
>
> Choose a situation from your placement and ask yourself:
>
> - What was my role in this situation?
> - Did I feel comfortable or uncomfortable? Why?
> - What actions did I take?
> - How did I and others act?
> - Was it appropriate?
> - How could I have improved the situation for myself, the patient, my mentor?
> - What can I change in future?
> - Do I feel as if I have learnt anything new about myself?
> - Did I expect anything different to happen? What and why?
> - Has it changed my way of thinking in any way?
> - What knowledge from theory and research can I apply to this situation?
> - What broader issues, for example ethical, political or social, arise from this situation?
> - What do I think about these broader issues?

and find myself not using them so formally, more as a checklist ... Reflection becomes increasingly intuitive and creative. However, for the novice reflective practitioner having worked through the MSR cues, take a pause and take a further step backwards from the text to see the bigger picture.' (Johns 2009, p.74)

The MSR has emerged from Chris John's extensive work through which practitioners have explored their experiences in supervision. His work is well loved and well known in nursing, and across other disciplines, and is certainly worthy of further reading.

Reflective Framework (Stephenson 1994)

This framework emerged from the student experiences of Sarah Stephenson, who wrote in the first edition of this book. Sarah was one of the first graduates from our programme and was immersed in reflection throughout her undergraduate studies. Stephenson's framework remains pertinent to contemporary practice, is well liked by students for its utility and particularly encourages them to broaden their thinking in relation to practice (Box 9.3). As a result, her framework remains worth sharing with others and is included in our undergraduate professional assessment document at Oxford Brookes University. I have used Stephenson's framework

Chapter 9

with students reflecting on their clinical experiences; they have found it a useful and challenging guide to reflective tutorial groups and so have I!

Typology of Reflection: dimensions and guiding questions (adapted from Jay and Johnson 2002)

Finally, Jay and Johnson (2002) have outlined dimensions of reflection and useful guiding questions that have been adapted here to provide another valuable framework for reflection in nursing (Box 9.4). They originally developed this as a typology to guide teacher educators in teaching reflection to preservice teachers in the USA. They used this as an outline for discourse between individuals and groups so that experience could be articulated and examined. They were very clear that it provides a supportive scaffolding for learning the process of reflection and thus it is not to be viewed as a series of restrictive steps. Whilst it does not emphasise the affective side of reflection in a way that other frameworks do, it does provide a structure that I could see would be useful for nurses, and one which again encourages broader thinking, and thus I have adapted it with this in mind.

Key messages about frameworks for reflection

My experience tells me that the Reflective Cycle is particularly favoured by many undergraduate students, with more complex frameworks often being adopted by higher degree students. The key factor seems to be finding something that helps you to get started and that eventually gives you the confidence to, as Bolton (2001) suggested, deconstruct your own practice. All of these frameworks have strengths and limitations and more research exploring their use in practice, both clinical and educational, would be welcome. Remember that frameworks do not encompass all that reflection is or could be; you need to invest in developing the sorts of skills outlined above, think about the influences of good facilitation on reflection and take a look at the literature on reflection to get your own critical feel for it.

Finding someone to reflect with

Dialogue is essential in order to support as well as to challenge thinking (Clouder and Sellars 2004; Johns 2004) since without dialogue with others in order to nurture criticality, the reflective process can easily slip into non-critical self-affirmation (Bulman 2009). Quoting one of her own colleagues, Riddell (2007, p.122) likened the process of asking someone to question their assumptions to 'asking a goldfish to perceive water'; this highlights the importance of critical questioning in order to identify assumptions and examine beliefs and actions. Morgan and Johns (2005) have emphasised the importance of dialogue to the process of reflection

Box 9.4   Typology of Reflection: dimensions and guiding questions (Adapted from Jay and Johnson 2002 by Bulman.)

Below you will find three dimensions of reflection as described by Jay and Johnson. Each has a set of guiding questions which may be useful for reflecting on an experience or issue from your practice.

Describe the experience/matter for reflection (Descriptive Reflection)

- What happened?
- What worked well and for whom? How do I know?
- How did I and am I feeling?
- What am I pleased or concerned about?
- What do I not understand?
- Does any of this relate to my objectives for practice? To what extent are my objectives being met?

Reframe the experience/issue for reflection in the light of other views and evidence (Comparative Reflection)

- What are other views on what happened? How do other people directly or indirectly involved describe and explain what happened?
- How does research contribute to my understanding?
- How can I improve what is not working well for me?
- If I have an objective, what other ways are there to accomplish it?
- How do others accomplish the same objective?
- When I look at other perspectives and alternatives, who is served and who is not?

Having considered implications, establish a renewed perspective (Critical Reflection)

- What are the implications of the experience/issue when viewed from alternative perspectives?
- Given these alternatives and their implications and my own morals/ethics, which are most useful to understand this particular experience/issue better?
- What does the experience/issue reveal about the purposes of nursing?
- What does the experience/issue reveal about the moral and political dimensions of nursing?
- How does this reflective process inform and renew my perspectives?

and research studies reiterate this; for instance, Graham (2000) and Olofsson (2005) highlight the importance of sharing experiences of working with patients and how nurses value the opportunity to talk. Paterson and Zderad's (1988) seminal work on humanistic nursing has acknowledged that the expression of nursing dialogue is not easy, yet nurses need to find ways to do this. Therefore, it is necessary to consider how you can get into dialogue in order to challenge and develop your practice. This could be with a mentor, clinical supervisor, critical friend or reflective buddy, the point being that it is this process that can help to develop your critique of practice.

The oral tradition in nursing has most notably been described by Street (1992) in her well-known critical ethnographic study of the oral culture that dominates and is maintained by nurses. She suggested that nurses do not have a tradition that supports the recording of data about their practice and so this impoverishes nursing, because this knowledge is then overlooked. Indeed, participants in her study suggested that it was a luxury for nurses to take time to sit and think about practice issues, so that nurses were not encouraged to talk and write about their nursing. Street suggested that such a culture was related to oppression, creating circumstances where nurses were not able collaboratively to critique their practice. This meant that nurses were unable to challenge the dominant medical and administrative culture perpetuated through means of written communication. Whilst the 'scientific' voice of medicine continues to remain dominant in healthcare for many reasons, it could be said that medical practice is also not based on scientific or propositional knowledge alone. Amongst other issues, the medical voice is strong because doctors have been educated to express their practice confidently in a way that, in the past, nurses have not. So we, as nurses, also need to find ways to articulate and communicate our practice and reflective dialogue offers a useful route.

A reflective colleague, mentor or supervisor can provide a sounding board, open up different perspectives and provide support and guidance. It is helpful to find someone who already has experience of using reflection and who is someone that you trust, if you are going to share and explore your experiences and feelings. This facilitative role cannot be ignored in the reflective process because as I have said, it is so easy to slip into non-critical self-affirmation without it. There are those who criticise this aspect of reflection as more akin to surveillance, confession and correction (e.g. Pryce 2002; Rolfe and Gardner 2006). This is provocative reading which misses the spirit of reciprocity and curiosity that should be part of reflective colleagues skillfully helping practitioners to see the effects of their practice. Yet it highlights the need to continually critique the development of coaching and facilitation so as not to lose sight of the motivation behind it, which is to *critically explore practice in order to make a positive difference to people in need of nursing.*

Reflective discussion with colleagues is something that is almost taken for granted or not given the prominence that it deserves (see Chapter 6 on clinical supervision). Some people have reflective buddies or clinical supervisors with whom they regularly discuss their practice; this is becoming more difficult to achieve in challenging times for healthcare and education. Positive work environments can also foster a climate where challenge is expected but supportive discussion is also encouraged. This type of discussion may not be labelled reflection by purists but is part of the process of enquiry in order to move on one's thinking and practice; it is also affected by staffing levels in the current climate. The key thing is to reflect with people you respect and whose opinion you value and to find an environment where you can be up for a challenge.

Developing your reflective writing

Now a few condensed tips on the key issues in developing your reflective writing. Essentially, keeping a regular diary is extremely useful, since the memory of events can fade quickly, even for those with the most photographic of memories. It is helpful to build up a record of your personal repertoire of experience in a diary which you will be able to use to reflect back on and draw from. It is worth setting aside time to write in your diary in a form that feels comfortable for you. You can record experiences concerning situations that seemed dramatic or special in practice (don't forget to preserve anonymity and confidentiality). However, it is possible to miss out on seemingly routine or mediocre events which, on reflection, could prove to be useful learning experiences. Diary keeping requires motivation and commitment; some people find it suits them and others just don't get along with it. The most important thing is to find a method of contemplating your experiences that works for you. Sylvina Tate offers some wonderfully detailed tips to help you with diary keeping and writing in Chapter 3.

Educationalists should be aware of the support and guidance needed if diary keeping or journal writing is to be advocated as part of learning about practice. They need to consider how writing about experience is shared and supported, if students are asked to keep journals. The work of Thorpe (2004) and Appleton (2008), amongst others, are worthy of scrutiny before students are exposed to the rigours of diary or journal keeping.

Some practical tips on writing

Writing is something we all have to work at. The tips below are included to help with this and were generated and adapted from focus group work (Bulman and Burns 2000) with some generous-hearted postregistration students who were developing their own reflective writing and didn't mind sharing some of their experiences.

1. Use a reflective framework – keep it near to where you study; refer to it as you work on your first jottings.
2. Get something down on paper as early as possible, not necessarily something academic or part of assessed work but something you can check out with your mentor, clinical supervisor, critical friend or reflective buddy in the first instance.
3. Try to discipline yourself to keep a regular reflective diary; write down what happened and why. Ask, what did I learn and what would I do next time?
4. Look back over your diary – use it to inform the academic work required of you.
5. Make sure you fix up an early meeting with your mentor, clinical supervisor, critical friend or reflective buddy – and keep it! Check s/he knows what is expected of you and her/him.
6. Be aware of the repertoire of experience you develop. You can draw on and store up experiences that you could use later in your reflective work, by making notes and jotting things down so that important experiences are not lost.
7. Get to know your mentor, clinical supervisor, critical friend or reflective buddy; use opportunities for reflective conversations.
8. If you can, get to know your teacher; make the most of any individual or group opportunities to get feedback on any assessed reflection.
9. Write down some reflection, then leave it for a while (about 2 days); you may find it easier to be critical on your return.
10. If you are using a framework, refer to it and ensure all stages are covered in order to complete your analysis.
11. Go deep, not wide in your analysis.
12. Live with lack of perfection; realise you won't always achieve the ideal, so do what you can with some sense of direction.
13. Seek out colleagues who support you.

Reading examples of reflective writing is also valuable to get an idea of how other people have gone about it. You will be able to go back through this book and find some which will be helpful to you in almost every chapter. For other good and varied examples of reflection, I would also recommend looking at Bulman and Schutz (2004, 2008), Bolton (2005), Johns and Freshwater (2005) and Johns (2009).

Included below are two edited examples kindly donated by second-year undergraduate adult nursing students who wrote an assignment exploring challenging issues in their practice – in both these cases they have considered the challenges involved in caring for patients with dementia. These two examples will give you an insight into student nurses' stories about their practice and hopefully show how the process of reflection can be uncomfortable, yet can encourage analytical thinking and open-mindedness about practice, as well as a motivation to develop practice for the better. Of course, there will be things that the writing does not capture; for example, it isn't possible to show the development of reflection through a couple of examples, nor do they reveal all the contextual information that allowed these students to reflect on their experiences. These are things that you need to experience and think about for yourself with support from mentors, teachers and colleagues.

As you read these examples think about:

- how different stages and features of these examples would fit into the reflective frameworks above
- how the students have interpreted reflection.
- how these examples demonstrate different aspects of caring for patients with dementia and illustrate the 'swampy lowlands' of practice problems
- whether these examples resonate with your own experiences in practice
- what new knowledge you think the students have gained from their reflection.

Example 1

Includes extracts from a student's reflection on a patient with dementia and her encounter with a care support worker.

'... I was feeding a patient who was in bed and had been very ill. In the bed next to her was another patient who had dementia (Mrs M) ... Mrs M was able to mobilise using a Zimmer frame quite safely and independently (she had no history of falls), although she was quite slow. Mrs M was often disorientated of place and time and was slightly deaf. On this particular occasion she had begun quietly talking to herself and had expressed concern that her children needed picking up and that she would have to go and collect them. As I was in the middle of feeding someone who often declined to have anything to eat and was malnourished, I felt my priority was to make sure she had as much to eat as possible before she fell asleep again. For this reason, I didn't go over to Mrs M and didn't want to address her by loudly speaking over the patient whom I was feeding at the time.

Mrs M stood up and started to arrange some of her belongings on the bed. At this point a care support worker (CSW) had arrived and stood close to Mrs M with her arms crossed. The CSW frowned and asked Mrs M what she was doing. Mrs M said that she was getting ready to go and pick her children up. The CSW told Mrs M that her children did not need picking up and that she was confused. The CSW told Mrs M to sit down. Mrs M raised her voice and insisted that her children needed collecting, and that she would have to do it as there was nobody else. The CSW told Mrs M that she couldn't leave and needed to stay on the ward so the staff could look after her. Mrs M then went on to express frustration that no-one would listen to her and that she was being kept prisoner against her will. The conversation soon became a repetitive cycle and continued for several minutes.

Mrs M became more animated as the conversation went on. I said to the CSW "you've tried, maybe just leave it now". She turned to look at me and frowned, and continued to exchange words with Mrs M, disagreeing with everything she said. The situation had become quite uncomfortable, both for myself and other patients in the bay, who had looked at me expressing disapproval for what was happening. I said again to the CSW, "I think maybe you should just leave it, you're winding her up". The CSW strongly objected to my comment by saying I didn't know what I was talking about. She said to me: "Who do you think you are telling me what to do?". The CSW continued to verbally express to me how inappropriate she regarded my comment. The CSW asked me what I would do differently that would be so much better. I said "I wasn't saying I could have done better, all I meant was sometimes it's better to just leave things to calm down and come back later". She then left the bay, still speaking at me very loudly as she left.

When I finished feeding the patient I spent some time talking to Mrs M. After she had calmed down I continued with the remaining tasks I was yet to complete: shaving two male patients. After this I shared my negative feelings with another student nurse. I then found a quiet room and wrote down what had happened and how I was feeling. I also spent the rest of the shift avoiding the CSW. When I finished the placement several weeks later I raised concern by discussing the experience with my link lecturer and academic advisor.

I experienced a number of negative emotions during and after this event. I was saddened, disappointed and annoyed at the CSW for not having any patience for Mrs M. I believe the CSW treated Mrs M with a lack of respect and failed to put her well-being first. I felt a degree of anger towards the CSW for having a lack of self-awareness and seemingly being unwilling to consider the effect of her actions or adopt an alternative approach. I was also angry on behalf of Mrs M who didn't have her concerns validated or her needs met. I felt that her dignity had not been preserved as she was made to feel foolish. After my attempts to improve the situation had failed, I also felt helpless to change what was happening. I was frustrated at having such little power or respect as a student nurse. My self-esteem had taken a big hit too. Furthermore I felt shaken up and was highly stressed.

After the adrenaline in my system had worn off I started to look at what happened under a new light. I did this by trying to appreciate things from not only Mrs M's point of view but also the CSW's. This was an attempt at positive reframing although it resulted in partial self-blame; an emotion-based (coping) strategy (Burgess *et al.* 2010). Another emotion-based coping strategy I used was to verbally vent to someone else. I tried to lessen the negative feelings associated with the challenging issue, after I had failed to change what was happening. Burgess *et al.* (2010) report that venting is a highly effective vehicle for stress reduction. Although this study is specific to an ICU setting, the significance of the findings on coping strategies are relevant to the wider field of nursing, as it relates to stressful situations in general.

Finally, I exhibited some avoidance-based behaviour by distracting myself from the stress I was feeling afterwards with other tasks. To some extent I was denying it had happened to me as I avoided further contact with the CSW. The fact that I was on my own in confronting the CSW added to my list of stressors. Vedhara *et al.* (2000) report that social support throughout a potentially stressful time can help reduce the amount of stress experienced by the individual. I further tried to alleviate my stress by writing about what had happened. As well as being a useful coping strategy, writing about such incidences also promotes self-awareness (Rungapadiachy 1999).

… Although I didn't feel I'd witnessed unsafe practice, I read the guidelines on caring for the older person (Nursing and Midwifery Council 2009) and felt I was right to raise the concern. After then reading the NMC (2010) guidance on raising and escalating concerns, I decided to raise the concern with my link lecturer. I felt unable to do this until I had completed the placement, however, as I feared it would have a negative impact on my relationships with the staff and remaining time on the ward. Such reluctance of students to report bad practice is illustrated in a study by Bellefontaine (2009). This qualitative study involves semi-structured interviews with six student nurses on clinical placements. Four main themes were identified in the analysis which contributed towards students not speaking out: the student–mentor relationship; actual or potential support provided by both the practice area and university; students' own personal confidence and professional knowledge base; and fear of failing clinical placements. Bellefontaine acknowledges that there is limited evidence but estimates that the types of worries experienced by myself are extremely common among student nurses on placement.

Rungapadiachy argues that an ability to act appropriately on what one finds is the result of developing high levels of self-awareness. Self-awareness is fundamental to good nursing practice. According to Jack and Smith (2007), 'being self-aware enables us to identify our strengths and also those areas that can be developed' (p.40). The awareness we have about ourselves continuously shapes our future development and requires us 'to stand outside of ourselves,

Chapter 9

reflect on ourselves and evaluate our intra- and interpersonal elements' (Rungapadiachy 1999, p.20).

On reflection, I could have been more assertive with what I said to the CSW, avoiding the criticism "you're winding her up". Since examining this incident I have become more aware of how I may be perceived by others. I believe this will strongly enhance my future practice. I will continue to give more of a consideration to how I am approaching a challenge. I would like to have been able to calmly give an example of an alternative approach to the CSW. At the time I was unaware of the evidence concerning communication that exists. This has highlighted to me the importance of always research-ing the subject area of a placement. This way you can give your concerns a stronger voice by supporting them with firm evidence.

After conducting research for the purpose of this assignment, I have also considered that my personality may have an effect on my ability to cope. I have discovered that I successfully approach a chal-lenging situation with a predominantly problem-based approach, although I could develop a tendency to deal with the emotions that arise as a result of the threat, rather than deal with the threat itself. For this reason I must engage in regular reflection and self-evaluation in order to monitor my stress levels and how I am coping. I need to work on being more assertive, particularly with my choice of words. It is important that I learn how to communicate concerns in a non-threatening and non-personalised way. I also need to be more vocal when I am experiencing stress, and seek social support at an earlier stage if possible, instead of or in addition to venting about it afterwards.'

Example 2

Involves a student nurse reflecting on the events that followed the nega-tive nursing handover of a patient with dementia. The patient was described as a very aggressive and violent gentleman, who had physically and verbally abused a member of staff and distressed other clients on the ward.

'I felt this was a challenging situation because I was assigned to work with Mr Brown (pseudonym) alongside my mentor and I sensed that there was no system or strategy put in place to manage the situa-tion. During the handover, all the staff nurse did was describe and complain about the issue; there was no indication of an action plan established to manage or prevent Mr Brown's behaviour. My mentor reacted to the handover by listening to what the staff nurse had to say but did not question her on how to deal with the situation and just accepted the fact that we may have a difficult shift.

Following this handover and when first approaching Mr Brown to introduce ourselves (myself and my mentor), he did not acknowledge our presence. He did this by pretending to be asleep. My mentor responded to this behaviour by moving closer to Mr Brown, lowering herself down to his level to make eye contact with him and she gently placed her hand on top of his. She repeated "Good morning Mr Brown" and he opened his eyes, stared at both me and my mentor, and then closed his eyes again. By my mentor approaching Mr Brown in this way, she displayed confidence and was not intimidated by Mr Brown's reported behaviour towards other members of staff. I also adopted this attitude from my mentor and behaved in a manner that was non-judgemental. I felt very positive towards the care I delivered for Mr Brown and was reassured by my mentor as she felt I was developing a good relationship with him as he fully accepted my care.

The initial encounter with Mr Brown was a positive one. He accepted both me and my mentor's presence as he felt comfortable to allow my mentor to make physical contact with him (by placing her hands on his). This way of non-verbal communication quickly helped to establish some interaction between Mr Brown and my mentor. Approaching Mr Brown from the front, moving down to his level and establishing eye contact all helped to send a positive message to him, which resulted in a mutual respect being formed between all three of us. This, therefore, allowed me to feel at ease when caring for Mr Brown and provided me with confidence to develop a good therapeutic relationship with him.

The bad point of my experience was during the handover when the staff nurse was describing issues she felt Mr Brown had caused. Her judgemental attitude made me feel much taken aback and uncertain towards the quality of care provided to him. Feeling nervous and anxious at the thought of caring for Mr Brown was exacerbated by the lack of management or strategies put in place to deal with or prevent his aggressive behaviour.

The Alzheimer's Society (2010, p.1) highlights that "a person with dementia may be trying to interpret a world that no longer makes sense to them" as their brain is acknowledging information incorrectly. This can lead to frustration for both the healthcare professionals and the client, which may result in avoidance of interaction. I strongly believe that this was the case for Mr Brown. Nurses on the ward found his behaviour extremely challenging as his actions affected the ward routine and needed additional support, so he was classed as disruptive.

Other healthcare professionals clearly did have a different experience with Mr Brown compared to my own. In my opinion, this was because they believed that his behaviour was solely due to his condition and felt that there was nothing they could do to prevent or alleviate his behaviour. However, my mentor and I proved otherwise. The coping strategy we applied was effective communication.

Chapter 9

The Alzheimer's Society (2010) has developed a document entitled *Top Tips for Nurses* to guide them in the techniques to aid communication with a person with dementia. These include:

- maintaining eye contact
- approaching the client from the front
- minimising distractions
- being quiet and listening
- not patronising
- using short sentences
- speaking clearly and calmly.

I observed and adopted these techniques from my mentor, which resulted in Mr Brown's needs being met and prevented him from displaying aggressive behaviour towards me and my mentor.

Self-awareness was also key when coping with Mr Brown's potential disruptive behaviour. Thompson (2002) describes self-awareness as a process of understanding your own feelings, attitudes and beliefs and acknowledging how this may affect others. My mentor was very self-aware as she did not allow her colleague's previous experiences with Mr Brown to affect how she treated him. Knowing he had been physically abusive to another member of staff, she still approached Mr Brown with confidence and did not display any negative verbal and non-verbal communication. I have seen how effective good communication and self-awareness are as coping strategies and seen from the client's point of view how this can change their attitude towards healthcare professionals and how their care needs can be adequately met.

Person-centred care "must recognise individual differences and specific needs" (Department of Health 2001, p.23), particularly since dementia affects each person in a unique way. Kitwood (1997) proposed a collection of culturally grounded needs required for a person with dementia to help function as a respectable human being. These proposed needs are: giving and receiving of love, comfort, attachment, inclusion, occupation and identity.

In meeting as many of these needs as possible, nurses can help to maintain personhood when caring for a client with cognitive impairment (Dewing 2000). The 'This is Me' leaflet, produced by the Alzheimer's Society, aims to provide healthcare professionals with information about the client's likes, dislikes, routines and needs that are unique to them to enhance personalised care.

Effective care also acknowledges the need for families, or other individuals who have been involved in supporting the person with dementia at home, to input towards their care received in an acute setting (Department of Health 2010). Kitwood (1997) also stresses the importance of family involvement in the care of a person with dementia. This is because, according to Jootun and McGhee (2011), nurses can make quick judgements about a client with dementia, but by exploring their history it can help nurses to acknowledge aspects of the client's identity and wishes which may have been ignored (Morton 1999). So, understanding each individual can help to predict or prevent disturbing behaviour. All behaviour is a form of communication and it is important to note that disruptive behaviour is not always due to the person with dementia's condition. Dean (2011) states that people with dementia can cause disturbances on the ward because they frequently are not given adequate pain relief.

Price (2006) does argue how realistic is it to provide person-centred care for a person with dementia, focusing on the person's holistic needs as well as their physical needs. This is supported by the Royal College of Nursing which discovered that nurses are prevented from providing adequate care in meeting a person with dementia's holistic needs because their workload is too great and staffing is too low (Dean 2011). However, by not taking the long-term approach into trying to find out why the client is displaying disruptive behaviour, for example, this itself can increase the nursing team workload.

In caring for Mr Brown following the poor handover, I have learnt that effective communication is the key to help establish a therapeutic relationship with a dementia client. By reflecting on my experience it has helped to reinforce the techniques used to enhance communication with a person with dementia but has also enabled me to gain evidence-based knowledge of these techniques. I have been able to take into account the client's viewpoint, for example, reasons for disruptive behaviour, but also look at the healthcare professional's point of view as to reasons why dementia care may be inadequate, i.e. high workload and insufficient or inappropriate training.

I have also learnt that I do have good communication skills with clients, which I shall continue to enhance with further practice placement experience. I have also learnt that I need to question healthcare practice more and to do this I need to continue to enhance my evidence-based knowledge. For example, if I were aware of the 'This is Me' guide or the 'Let's respect' campaign, I would have asked to see information on these and if not available find out reasons as to why.

A broader recommendation I would make to enhance good-quality nursing practice based on my critical reflection of my challenging experience is education and training. During my assignment, the nurses assumed that the client's aggressive behaviour was entirely due to his condition. However, by carrying out my reflection I have learnt that this behaviour may have been a form of him communicating his frustration to the nurses in not meeting and understanding his needs. Therefore, if nurses felt confident and competent in working with this client group they may have acknowledged that there may be underlying issues causing the client's behaviour, reinforcing person-centred care.'

Chapter 9

Reading the literature

This book and past editions should provide you with some useful background on reflection, and there are many other books and articles on reflection in nursing and other disciplines that you will find helpful. You just need to take a look at what is out there. From a broader perspective, I would also recommend McCarthy and Rose's (2010) book on values-based health and social care, Bonis' (2009) concept analysis of knowing in nursing, Wackerhausen's (2009) and Clark's (2009) perspectives on inter-professional collaboration for challenging and developing constructive reflection, Kinsella's (2007) deeper look at Schön's theory of reflective practice and Tanner's (2009) editorial on evidence-based practice, critical thinking and clinical judgement. Basically, I want to encourage you to read broadly in order to develop a wide appreciation of opinions, issues and evidence, and as a result to begin to establish an idea of what you personally find helpful in starting to reflect.

Having the courage to change and challenge

As I have highlighted earlier in the chapter, having the courage to change and challenge is not easy and the current social, political and cultural climate within healthcare and higher education makes this demanding for nurses. One of the things I encourage my own students to do is to consider ways in which they can develop their assertiveness skills, as I have found assertiveness training a useful adjunct in my own practice and in life. Perhaps you are fortunate to work in an environment where positive change and constructive challenge are welcomed in the workplace, and then it is easier to be brave and voice your reflections on practice. If you are not in this position, you need to seek out supportive and facilitative networks, before you set off on a reflective pathway (see Chapter 1 for more thoughts on this). Whatever the situation, contemporary nursing needs effective and person-centred nurses who can articulate their professional knowledge to others, develop meaningful practice, liberate their learning, and consequently make an active, positive difference to patient care.

Conclusion

This final chapter offers some condensed assistance in 'getting started' on your journey with reflection. It complements and summarises key considerations and critiques concerning reflection presented throughout this book. It highlights some issues to contemplate at the beginning of the journey and presents some key suggestions as you begin your journey with reflection. These suggestions encompass skills for reflection, reflective frameworks, the value of finding someone to reflect with, developing your writing, reading literature on reflection as well as more broadly, and having the courage to change and challenge. Reflection has something to offer nurses and I know it is a concept that nurses continue to be interested in. We hope that this book provides you with some inspiration to start out on your own journey.

References

Alzheimer's Society (2010) *Top Tips for Nurses*. Available at: www.alzheimers.org. uk/site/scripts/documents_info.php?documentID=1211

Appleton, J.M. (2008) Using reflection in a palliative care education programme. In: Bulman, C. and Schutz, S. (eds) *Reflective Practice in Nursing. The Growth of the Professional Practitioner*, 4th edn. Blackwell, Oxford.

Bellefontaine, N. (2009) Exploring whether student nurses report poor practice they have witnessed on placements. *Nursing Times*, **105**(35), 28–31.

Bolton, G. (2001) *Reflective Practice. Writing and Professional Development*. Paul Chapman Publishing, London.

Bolton, G. (2005). *Reflective Practice: Writing and Professional Development*, 2nd edn. Sage, London.

Bonis, S.A. (2009) Knowing in nursing: a concept analysis. *Journal of Advanced Nursing*, **65**(6), 1328–1341.

Borton, T. (1970) *Reach, Touch and Teach*. Hutchinson, London.

Bulman, C. (2009) Constructing reflection in nursing: a qualitative exploration of reflection through a post-registration palliative care programme. Unpublished PhD thesis, University of Southampton, School of Health Sciences.

Bulman, C. and Burns, S. (2000) Students' perspectives on reflective practice. In: Burns, S. and Bulman, C. (eds) *Reflective Practice. The Growth of the Professional Practitioner*, 2nd edn. Blackwell Science, Oxford.

Bulman, C. and Schutz, S. (2004) *Reflective Practice in Nursing*, 3rd edn. Blackwell Science, Oxford.

Bulman, C. and Schutz, S. (2007) Practical wisdom in professional practice. Contemplating some of the issues. Paper presented at the Creating Phronesis Conference, June, Aalborg, Denmark.

Bulman, C. and Schutz, S. (2008) *Reflective Practice in Nursing. The Growth of the Professional Practitioner*, 4th edn. Blackwell, Oxford.

Burgess, L., Irvine, F. and Wallymahmed, A. (2010) Personality, stress and coping in intensive care nurses: a descriptive exploratory study. *Nursing in Critical Care*, **15**(3), 129–140.

Burnard, P. (2005). Reflections on reflection (editorial). *Nurse Education Today*, **25**, 85–86.

Burns, S. and Bulman, C. (eds) (2000) *Reflective Practice. The Growth of the Professional Practitioner*, 2nd edn. Blackwell Science, Oxford.

Clark, P.G. (2009) Reflecting on reflection in interprofessional education: Implications for theory and practice. *Journal of Interprofessional Care*, **23**(3), 213–223.

Clouder, L. and Sellars, J. (2004). Reflective practice and clinical supervision: an interprofessional perspective. *Journal of Advanced Nursing*, **46**(3), 262–269.

Dean, E. (2011) Dementia care impeded by workloads. *Nursing Standard*, **25**(35), 15.

Department of Health (2001) *National Service Framework for Older People.* Available at: www.dh.gov.uk/prod_consum_dh/groups/dh_digitalassets/@dh/@en/documents/digitalasset/dh_4071283.pdf

Dewing, J. (2000) Promoting wellbeing in older people with cognitive impairment. *Elderly Care*, **12**(4), 19–22.

Driscoll, J. (1994) Reflective practice for practice – a framework of structured reflection for clinical areas. *Senior Nurse*, **14**(1), 47–50.

Driscoll, J. (ed) (2007) *Practising Clinical Supervision: A Reflective Approach for Healthcare Professionals.* Baillière Tindall/Elsevier, Edinburgh.

Eisner, E.W. (1991) *The Enlightened Eye: Qualitative Inquiry and the Enhancement of Educational Practice.* Macmillan, New York.

Gibbs, G., Farmer, B. and Eastcott, D. (1988) *Learning by Doing. A Guide to Teaching and Learning Methods.* Far Eastern University, Birmingham Polytechnic, Birmingham.

Graham, I.W. (2000). Reflective practice and its role in mental health nurses' practice development: a year long study. *Journal of Psychiatric and Mental Health Nursing*, **7**, 109–117.

Jack, K. and Smith, A. (2007) Promoting self-awareness in nurses to improve nursing practice. *Nursing Standard*, **21**(32), 47–52.

James, C.R. and Clarke, B.A. (1994) Reflective practice in nursing: issues and implications for nursing education. *Nurse Education Today*, **14**, 82–90.

Jay, J.K. and Johnson, K.L. (2002) Capturing complexity: a typology of reflective practice for teacher education. *Teaching and Teacher Education*, **18**, 73–85.

Johns, C. (2000) *Becoming a Reflective Practitioner. A Reflective and Holistic Approach to Clinical Nursing, Practice Development and Clinical Supervision.* Blackwell Science, Oxford.

Johns, C. (2004) *Becoming a Reflective Practitioner*, 2nd edn. Blackwell, Oxford.

Johns, C. (2009) *Becoming a Reflective Practitioner*, 3rd edn. Wiley-Blackwell, Oxford.

Johns, C. and Freshwater, D. (2005) *Transforming Nursing Through Reflective Practice.* Blackwell Publishing, Oxford.

Jootun, D. and McGhee, G. (2011) Effective communication with people who have dementia. *Nursing Standard*, **25**(25), 40–46. Available at: http://nursingstandard.rcnpublishing.co.uk/resources/archive/GetArticleById.asp?ArticleId=8347

Kinsella, E.A (2007) Technical rationality in Schön's reflective practice: dichotomous or non-dualistic epistemological position. *Nursing Philosophy*, **8**, 102–113.

Kitwood, T. (1997) On being a person. In: Kitwood, T. (ed) *Dementia Reconsidered: The Person Comes First.* Open University Press, Milton Keynes, pp.7–19.

Kolb, D.A. (1984*) Experiential Learning – Experience as the Source of Learning and Development.* Prentice-Hall, New Jersey.

Mantzoukas, S. and Jasper, M.A. (2004) Reflective practice and daily ward reality: a covert power game. *Journal of Clinical Nursing*, **13**, 913–924.

McCarthy, J. and Rose, P. (2010) *Values-Based Health and Social Care: Beyond Evidence Based Practice.* Sage Publications, London.

Morgan, R. and Johns, C. (2005) The beast and the star: resolving contradictions within everyday practice. In: Johns, C. and Freshwater, D. (eds) *Transforming Nursing Through Reflective Practice.* Blackwell Publishing, Oxford.

Morton, I. (1999) *Person-Centred Approaches to Dementia Care.* Winslow, Oxford.

Nursing and Midwifery Council (2009) *Guidance for the Care of Older People.* Nursing and Midwifery Council, London.

Nursing and Midwifery Council (2010) *Raising and Escalating Concerns: Guidance for Nurses and Midwives.* Nursing and Midwifery Council, London.

Olofsson, B. (2005) Opening up: psychiatric nurses' experiences of participating in reflection groups focusing on the use of coercion. *Journal of Psychiatric and Mental Health Nursing,* **12**, 259–267.

Paterson, J.G. and Zderad, L.T. (1988) *Humanistic Nursing.* National League for Nursing, New York.

Powell, J. (1998) Reflection and the evaluation of experience. In: McMahon, R. and Pearson, A. (eds) *Nursing as Therapy,* 2nd edn. Stanley Thornes, London.

Price, B. (2006) Exploring person-centred *care Nursing Standard,* **20**(50), 49–56. Available at: http://nursingstandard.rcnpublishing.co.uk/resources/archive/GetArticleById.asp?ArticleId=4487

Pryce, A. (2002) Refracting experience: reflection, post modernity and transformations. *Nursing Times Research,* **7**(4), 298–310.

Riddell, T. (2007) Critical assumptions: thinking critically about critical thinking. *Journal of Nursing Education,* **46**(3), 121–126.

Rolfe, G. and Gardner, L. (2006) 'Do not ask who I am …' Confession, emancipation and (self)-management through reflection. *Journal of Nursing Management,* **14**, 593–600.

Rungapadiachy, D.M. (1999) *Interpersonal Communication and Psychology for Health Care Professionals.* Butterworth Heinemann, Oxford.

Schön, D.A. (1983) *The Reflective Practitioner.* Basic Books, San Francisco.

Schön, D.A. (1987) *Educating the Reflective Practitioner.* Jossey-Bass, San Francisco.

Smith, P. and B. Gray (2001) Reassessing the concept of emotional labour in student nurse education: role of link lecturers and mentors in a time of change. *Nurse Education Today,* **21**, 230.

Stephenson, S. (1994) Reflection – a student's perspective. In: Palmer, A., Burns, S. and Bulman, C. (eds) *Reflective Practice: The Growth of the Professional Practitioner.* Blackwell Science, Oxford.

Street, A.F. (1992) *Inside Nursing: A Critical Ethnography of Clinical Nursing Practice.* State University of New York Press, New York.

Tanner, C.A. (2009) The case for cases: a pedagogy for developing habits of thought. (Editorial) *Journal of Nursing Education,* **48**(6), 299–300.

Thompson, N. (2002) *People Skills,* 2nd edn. Palgrave Macmillan, Basingstoke.

Thorpe, K. (2004) Reflective learning journals: from concept to practice. *Reflective Practice,* **5**(3), 327–343.

Vedhara, K., Addy, L. and Wharton, L. (2000) The role of social support as a moderator of the acute stress response: in situ versus empirically associations. *Psychology and Health,* **15**, 297–307.

Wackerhausen, S. (2009) Collaboration, professional identity and reflection across boundaries. *Journal of Interprofessional Care,* **23**(5), 455–473.

Chapter 9

Index

Reflective Practice in Nursing, Fifth Edition. Edited by Chris Bulman and Sue Schutz.
© 2013 John Wiley & Sons, Ltd. Published 2013 by John Wiley & Sons, Ltd.